The Breast Connection

A Laywoman's Guide
To the Treatment of Breast Disease
By Chinese Medicine

by
Honora Lee Wolfe

with a Preface by
Bob Flaws

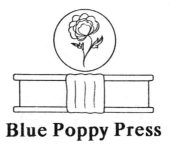

Blue Poppy Press

PUBLISHED BY:

BLUE POPPY PRESS
1775 LINDEN AVE.
BOULDER, CO 80304

FIRST EDITION
MAY, 1989

ISBN 0-936185-13-9

Printed at Westview Press, Boulder, CO
Cover printed at D & K Printing, Boulder, CO

ACKNOWLEDGEMENTS

For their editorial and moral support, I wish to thank Nina Yanowitch, M. Marie Morris, and Christine Covert. For his continued inspiration and unstinting pursuit of excellence, I am most grateful to my husband, Bob Flaws.

PREFACE

It is with great joy that I have the opportunity to introduce this book on the traditional Chinese prevention and treatment of breast disease by Honora Lee Wolfe. As my wife, Honora has travelled with me step for step the path of Chinese medicine. It was Honora who introduced me to Dr. (Eric) Tao Xi-yu and Michael Broffman, my two first Chinese medical mentors. I put my first acupuncture needles in on her. Honora helped to compile and co-author *Prince Wen Hui's Cook; Chinese Dietary Therapy*, and she has edited and designed all of Blue Poppy Press' publications. At the same time, she has gone to China to study at the Shanghai College of Traditional Chinese Medicine three times while being a mother, a housewife, and our clinic's business manager. Whatever I have personally been able to accomplish as a practitioner and writer on Chinese medicine I owe to my wife's continuous support and now I could not be happier that she has become a practitioner of this art in her own right.

In the following book, Ms. Wolfe has attempted to explain to the modern American layperson the mechanics of breast dysfunction and disease according to the logic of traditional Chinese medicine. Chinese medicine's description of the cause and mechanics of breast disease is logical and systematic. However, beyond its self-consistency and rationality, it is also eminently practical and efficient. Chinese medicine sees all breast disease as related. It describes a disease mechanism continuum, explaining why certain benign breast conditions evolve into malignant ones in some women. As such, traditional Chinese medicine can provide modern women with a logical map to help them avoid serious, life-threatening breast diseases through early Chinese medical treatment of related conditions and through modifications in diet, exercise, and lifestyle.

The map Chinese medicine paints of breast disease is easy to read and easy to follow once one entertains the possibility of the key propositions of traditional Chinese medicine. It is a map on which there are no unknown continents or trackless wildernesses. Honora Lee Wolfe has done a great service in making this map available to her sisters of all ages. It is both her and Blue Poppy's hope that this introduction for laywomen to the Chinese medical theory and treatment of breast disease may help lessen the number of Western women who will develop and suffer from these diseases.

Bob Flaws, DOM, CMT, Dipl.Ac.

TABLE OF CONTENTS

For my Mother, Martha Lee Wolfe
with love and gratitude.

INTRODUCTION

What's Wrong With This Picture?

From the onset of her period at age 13 Sarah had had severe menstrual cramps and swollen breasts. At age 25 she was diagnosed as having fibrocystic breasts and severe PMS; at 38 she had a benign cyst removed from her breast; at 47 a lumpectomy was performed on the same breast due to carcinoma in situ. Sarah died at age 55 from metastatic carcinoma of the breast. Why did this happen? Could it have been prevented?

Breast diseases are all too common among 20th century American women. More than half of all American women have some medical complaint concerning their breasts at some time during their lives. In a recent article appearing in *The Journal of Chinese Medicine*, Mazin Al-Khafaji states that 45 - 55% of all Western women will have palpable neoplasms (growths) of the breast.[1] Although only a small percentage of these will be life-threatening, such neoplasms can be both painful and frightening, thus affecting other aspects of a woman's life as well.

For most women, breast disease is a fearful topic. This is largely because the Western medical treatment of breast disease is not entirely satisfactory. Western medicine has few if any treatments to offer for the so-called benign breast diseases. And, while radical mastectomies have decreased and lumpectomies increased

1

in recent years for the treatment of malignancies, women still fear the possible invasion and mutilation of their bodies. Many are as frightened of the therapy as of the disease itself. The loss or disfigurement of a breast has a psychological and sexual self-image impact much larger than the actual physical experience.

Traditional Chinese medicine, on the other hand, has both a rational and humane theory about the causation and prevention of breast disease and effective treatments for most breast diseases. This is especially so when one understands that according to Chinese medicine, various diseases of the breast, are in fact, connected. They usually exist on a continuum and not as independent, isolated diseases. Because Chinese medicine can see and describe these connections, it can very effectively treat the beginning stages of this continuum, thus avoiding the later stages altogether. For women who are further along on this continuum, i.e. who have developed breast cancer, a combination of Western and traditional Chinese medicines is, perhaps, the most effective approach. However, if a woman understands the Chinese view concerning the cause and progression of breast disease she should be much better able to prevent any serious disease from arising.

This small book is an attempt to explain to American women the insights of traditional Chinese medicine concerning breast disease. It is offered in the hope that it may help alleviate some of the worry, pain, and suffering of women with breast disease by providing them with a clear explanation of their disease, possible preventive measures they might take, and logical treatment alternatives.

SECTION I

Western Medicine & Breast Disease

CHAPTER I

The Difference Between Modern Western & Traditional Chinese Medicine

Modern Western medicine is based on Western biological science. As such, it is a material description of the human body, and its diagnosis and treatment are limited to only that which can be seen, measured, and weighed. If something cannot be seen, measured, or weighed, for Western medicine it does not exist. As a material description of reality, Western medicine is highly perceptive, systematic, and logical. However, most people throughout human history have believed that there is more to life and the universe than just that which can be seen, measured, and weighed. In addition, modern Western medicine is only a little more than one hundred years old and is limited by its youth and potential for short-sightedness.

Traditional Chinese medicine is based on *both* a material and an energetic description of reality. And in Chinese medicine, relatively more attention is placed on describing the unseen, immaterial, energetic life-force called Qi^2 (pronounced chee) in Chinese. As a description of the energetic level of reality, Chinese medicine is equally perceptive, systematic, and logical. Although different from the Western medical description of health and disease, the Chinese map of our internal terrain and environment has much more energetic and qualitative detail. That is to say, Chinese medicine is a more complete and sophisticated medicine. This is so for several reasons:

1) With the possible exception of traumatic injuries, **energetic imbalances usually precede material ones**. Chinese medicine describes the energetic interactions within the body. It is these energetic interactions which produce/precede most changes in the material substances of the body. It is the *forte* of Western medicine to quantify and diagnose these more visible material changes. However, it is the energetic activity which, when proceeding correctly, produces health and balance. Conversely, if the energetic interactions of the body are interrupted or become unbalanced in any way, they eventually precipitate the occurrence of signs and symptoms. That is to say, energetic imbalances precede material ones. Chinese medicine can describe, diagnose, and treat these energetic imbalances in the body *before* they ever precipitate material changes which would be measurable by Western medical science.

2) **Chinese medical theory allows for preventive therapy.** Western medicine can diagnose and treat only dysfunction and disease of a material or physical nature. This means that the energetic process by which the disease has arisen must be already advanced enough to create an actual material or physical change in order for treatment to be given. Therefore, the emphasis of this style of medicine is remedial -- it is useful only after physical symptoms have arisen.

Chinese medicine, by contrast, can identify and treat an energetic imbalance before any material change can be measured. Moreover, because of Chinese medicine's rigorous and comprehensive theory, a good practitioner can often predict what will happen next in a given patient's disease process, and treat to stop the process before it begins or before it worsens. We will see

4

later that this ability to diagnose and treat preventively is extremely important in relationship to breast diseases.

3) **Chinese medicine is truly holistic.** The words holism and holistic have been bandied about a great deal over the last decade, often in relationship to medicine. According to *Webster's New World Dictionary* holism means, "A theory that the determining factors especially in living nature are irreducible wholes".[3] This is another way of saying that the parts of a living system reflect the whole and vice versa. Holistic medicine, therefore, should be a medicine which diagnoses & treats the whole person, and in which the meaning of each symptom presented relates to the whole in a meaningful and unfragmented way. Because it is based on atomistic reductionism, Western medicine is difficult to apply in this way, despite attempts by some M.D.'s who are not satisfied with the limitations of their medical system.

Chinese medical diagnostic procedure takes all the signs and symptoms which can be seen, heard or touched, and all symptoms which a person reports, and weaves them into a portrait of that person's internal landscape at that moment in time. Each sign or symptom can only be interpreted in relationship to all the others...that is, it only has meaning within the context of all the other signs or symptoms. Once the Chinese medical practitioner has painted this energetic "portrait" he or she must determine how this picture may change in relationship to the time of year, changes in the weather, the person's underlying constitution or tendencies, specific foods, sexual behavior, work, the menstrual cycle, or any other event (internal or external) which may in any way impact upon that person's energetic picture. Another way to say this is that Chinese medicine is holistic because it weaves a single, complete energetic fabric from the warp of its theory and woof of the patient's signs and symptoms, medical history, lifestyle and work conditions, the weather, season of the year, and everything else operating in that person's environment.

4) **Chinese medicine has stood the test of time.** Although it honors the words of Hippocrates and the lineages of Galen and Paracelsus, Western medicine is only just over a century old in its current form of practice, which really began with the theories of

Pasteur and Virchow. The longterm effects of many of its newer treatments and diagnostic techniques remain to be seen.

The professional literature and recorded clinical history of Chinese medicine span over two millennia. Although it has changed and grown over the centuries, as some of its more fringe or arcane theories and practices have been left behind, its basic theories have stood the test of time because they are based on natural laws which apply equally to human life and to "external" natural events. It is because of this unity with natural law that Chinese medicine is comprehensive yet simple, straightforward and yet profound.

Twentieth century Western culture has strayed far from natural law. We have polluted and abused our small and fragile planet almost beyond what it, or we, can healthily absorb. We have speeded up our communications and our travel. We have multiplied beyond comprehension the amount of information our minds must process each and every day. As Americans especially, we have complicated our lives and increased our background stress to the point where it is quite beyond our healthy carrying capacity. Our diseases -- medical, social, and environmental -- reveal this with little scrutiny. Perhaps this is why Chinese medicine is relevant to us now. Its truths have not deteriorated with time. In fact for those willing to look, their wisdom is all the more starkly revealed, in the light of our current medical and social predicament.

In relationship to breast disease specifically, the natural laws of Chinese medicine are applicable and timely. There is a clear theoretical description and diagnosis in each breast disease situation, and viable treatments as well. Before discussing this in detail, however, it may be useful for Western readers to see a short breakdown of the Western medical descriptions of the structure, function, and diseases of the breast.

CHAPTER II

The Structure & Function
Of The Breast
According To Western Biology

Knowledge of the structure and function of the healthy breast can go a long way toward relieving a woman's worry about breast disease. If a woman is aware of what normal breast tissue feels and looks like and what changes are normal in the breast at various times in her life, she will not worry when these normal changes occur and will be better able to recognize any abnormal changes.

The breast is composed of 15-25 lobes of glandular tissue which open into the nipple. These lobes are surrounded by fat which give the mass and smooth contour to the breast. Fibrous connective tissue called the Cooper's Ligament binds the breast together and provides support and protection for the glandular lobes.

Each lobe contains a duct system of lobules which is capable of conducting milk. The milk is produced by special cells called Acini Cells, and transported through the lobules to the nipple. These duct systems are rather like tributaries flowing into a river. These tributaries flow into a main reservoir directly behind the areola, the dark area surrounding the nipple. The milk can then flow from this reservoir to the surface of the nipple via another smaller system of ducts. The breasts are surrounded by lymph nodes which

7

help keep them free from infection. (See Figure 1.)

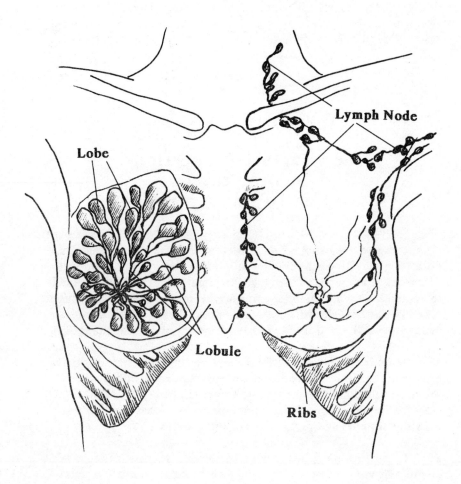

Figure 1.

On different women and at different times, breast tissue may variously feel soft, like fat tissue, or lumpy and thick, like glandular tissue. Women should get to know what is *normal for them* by doing regular breast self-examination. If a woman is not doing this simple procedure regularly, she should learn it and make it a non-discretionary part of her life each month. Most gynecologists, Planned Parenthood offices, women's clinics, and cancer research centers have pamphlets or videotapes explaining how to do a proper breast self-examination.

During periods of lactation, which is the sole *biological* function of the breast, the lobes will be larger, causing the breasts to expand in size. In most women, the breast is also highly erogenous, and responsive to sexual arousal. There may be changes in the color and texture of the skin of the breast during sexual activity, and the nipples will usually become very erect.

Other changes in the size and texture of the breast tissue during puberty, after the weaning of a child, and during menopause are regulated by the body's endocrine and lymphatic systems. After a period of lactation the breast may initially shrink to a smaller size than prior to pregnancy, then slowly return to a normal or even larger size than before. The breast tissue may also be softer than before. During menopause, the instability in the flow of hormones in the body may cause the breasts to increase even more in size. This increase may be temporary, or the breasts may remain larger until a woman is very old at which time the tissue of the breast becomes flaccid and the size of the breast again shrinks. These changes are all normal.[4]

CHAPTER III

Western Categories Of
Breast Disease
And Their Treatment

1) PREMENSTRUAL SYNDROME WITH BREAST DISTENTION AND PAIN

While premenstrual syndrome (PMS) is now a recognized category of dysfunction according to Western medicine, breast pain or distention by itself is not. For instance, there is no entry for breast distention and pain in the *Merck Manual of Diagnosis and Therapy* which is one of a Western doctor's most important desk references. It is, however, considered to be an important symptom in the PMS complex and is often a precursor of fibrocystic breast disease. For that reason, and because in Chinese medicine it is considered to be an extremely important symptom of imbalance, we will start with it here.

Dr. Niels H. Lauersen, in his book *PMS*, indicates that breast pain and distention are caused by hormonal changes (disturbances in the estrogen/progesterone levels) after ovulation and prior to menstruation each month.[5] Dr. Lauersen states that these changes are considered to be normal in most women. Since it is usually a self-limiting phenomenon related to the menses, it is rarely treated by Western medicine at all. Pain in the breast is not considered to be a common sign of breast cancer, but may be a sign of a breast cyst,[6] which is usually surgically removed.

2) FIBROCYSTIC BREAST DISEASE

As many as 30% of all American women may have this condition and it is the most common of all benign breast disorders. It usually occurs in women over 25, although new lumps rarely appear in post menopausal women. It is thought by Western medicine to be due to hormonal imbalance that can be triggered by a vast range of causes;[7] no one specific cause has been identified. This imbalance allows estrogen to predominate in the body and stimulates the growth of the glandular lobes and fibrous tissue of the breast, creating many small lumps and distention usually in the outer areas of the breast. The major symptom is visible swelling and pain with palpable lumpiness or thickening in the tissue. The lumps commonly come and go and the condition is usually worse during the week prior to menstruation when estrogen flow increases even more. (See Figure 2)

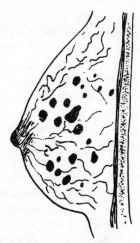

Figure 2.
Fibrocystic Lumps

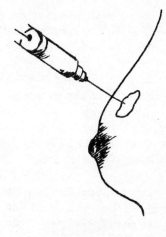

Figure 3.
Aspiration

12

Western medical treatment may include aspiration of the larger lumps. This is a procedure usually performed in a doctor's office, whereby a hypodermic needle is inserted directly into the lump to draw out any fluid. (See Figure 3)

In general, Western medicine does not consider it necessary to treat this condition. However, some Western research indicates that women with fibrocystic breast disease are three times more likely to develop breast cancer later in life than those without it.[8] Other Western medical sources say that no relationship exists between fibrocystic disease and breast cancer.

Western research also indicates that consumption of foods which contain large quantities of xanthines may worsen this condition.[9] Xanthines are found in coffee, black tea, cola drinks, chocolate, etc. Avoidance of these foods can reduce the problem significantly in many cases. A padded brassiere with good support is also suggested to help reduce pain and the heavy, distended sensation experienced during severe episodes since this reduces the movement of the breasts and protects them from external sources of irritation.[10]

In addition to aspiration, the one other Western medical treatment for fibrocystic disease is at this time still an experimental one. In a recent study done by Dr. Bernard A. Eskin of the Medical College of Pennsylvania and Dr. William A. Ghent of Queens University of Ontario, 100 mcg. of specially prepared elemental iodine was given daily to 143 women suffering from painful and fibrocystic breasts. Of all the cases, 72% experienced complete remission of symptoms, while another 27% had partial improvement. The remaining 1% had no change in their symptoms.[11] This treatment however, is not yet widely available or commonly recommended by Western gynecologists and it is unclear what, if any, consequences may exist from longterm iodine use at this dosage.

3) FIBROADENOMAS

This is the most common type of tumor seen in younger women and is considered to be the third most frequent of all breast diseases after fibrocystic disease and carcinoma of the breast. It is not malignant. The lump is firm, round, and moveable, like a marble under the skin. According to Western medicine, its cause is unknown. If it is painful or causes breast deformity, it is removed with local anesthesia. A fibroadenoma is not considered serious in itself, although its presence indicates the possibility of a higher risk for breast cancer later in life.[12] (See Figure 4)

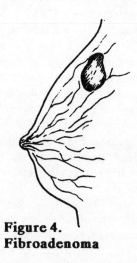

Figure 4.
Fibroadenoma

If a fibroadenoma breaks down of its own accord it can develop into what are called calcifications or microcalcifications. These are grainy calcium deposits developing as a breast cyst breaks down. Microcalcifications may or may not be associated with the development of breast cancer.

4) BREAST ABSCESSES (MASTITIS)

Due to local or systemic infection in the glands and ducts of the breast, this condition manifests as a painful, inflamed mass sometimes accompanied by discharge from the nipple. It is most commonly experienced after childbirth and during breastfeeding,

14

usually in a primapara (first time mother). When treated by Western medicine, breast feeding is often stopped and surgical drainage and/or antibiotics are administered.[13]

5) INTRADUCTAL PAPILLOMAS

These are very small tumors occurring in the terminal nipple ducts of the breast. They are frequently so small they are impossible to palpate. The main symptom is a serous, pinkish, or bloody discharge from the nipple. Treatment consists of surgical removal of the affected ducts and any other affected part of the breast. According to Western medicine, this tissue must be biopsied since a bloody discharge from the nipple can be due to malignancy especially if it occurs in only one breast.[14] (See Figure 5.)

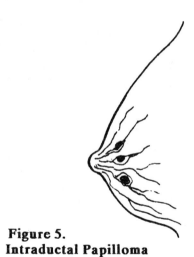

Figure 5.
Intraductal Papilloma

6) BREAST CANCER

Cancer of the breast is second only to lung cancer in frequency of occurrence in women. The American Cancer Society estimates

15

that in 1988 alone 135,000 new cases of this disease were diagnosed in the U.S. and that 42,300 women died of it.[15] Approximately one woman in 10 in this country will develop breast cancer at some point in her life at its present rate of occurrence. Carcinoma of the breast is the most common of all breast malignancies and carries with it the highest rate of mortality.[16] Signs of this disease include 1) a lump or thickening in the breast or armpit, 2) a change in the size or shape of the breast, 3) a bloody, brown, or green discharge from the nipple, and/or 4) a change in the color or texture of the skin of the breast of areola, such as dimpling, puckering, or scaliness. Pain is rarely a sign of breast cancer. According to Western medicine, the earlier breast cancer is detected and treated, the better are a woman's chance of complete recovery.

Western medical diagnosis of breast cancer is usually made by a combination of palpation (feeling the size, texture, and movability of a lump or thickening), aspiration (using a needle and syringe to withdraw fluid or tissue for biopsy), mammography (breast x-ray to reveal tumors which cannot be felt), and biopsy (removal of some or all of the lump to check for cancerous cells). Other tests such as ultrasonography or thermography may also be used.

Depending upon what stage of cancer is discovered, Western medical treatment may include lumpectomy, partial or radical mastectomy, chemotherapy, radiation therapy, or hormone therapy. Most treatment involves two or more of these, done in stages.[17]

According to Western medicine, the cause of breast cancer is unknown but some women seem to have higher risk than others for developing the disease. Factors include:

1. Age - There is a higher incidence in older women.

2. Family History - The risk doubles if a mother or sister has had the disease.

3. Personal History - A history of benign breast cysts, early onset of menstruation, late or no childbirths, or late

16

menopause.[18]

Recent Western research indicates that diet may also affect the chances of contracting some types of cancer. Breast cancer appears to be more likely to occur in women whose diet is high in fat, low in fiber, and who are generally overweight.[19]

Whatever the causes, *any* woman can get breast cancer and *all* women should do breast self-examination every month, get regular health check-ups, and see a primary health care practitioner if any abnormal changes occur.

Analysis and Critique
Of Western Categorization and Therapy
For Breast Diseases

Western medicine is physical medicine. It describes in great detail the material structure and interrelationships of the tissues, cells, and chemical constituents of the human body. Its treatments tend to be swift, heroic, and invasive. While this type of therapy has its strong points, it often causes side effects and it rarely deals with root causes of diseases, often being unable to detect them. Because of this, it offers little to a patient in terms of preventive measures, and even less in terms of useful explanations of how the disease process begins and what can be done to abort this process before it becomes life-threatening.

For most of the breast diseases listed above, the only Western medical therapy available is removal of palpable lumps by surgery or aspiration. Few preventive measures are offered and for some disorders no treatment is considered necessary. This is so despite the fact that some Western medical research indicates a higher incidence of breast cancer in women who have had other breast diseases. Western medicine finds no rational, theoretic link from one breast disease entity to the next.

17

In the following chapters I hope to fill these gaps in the Western medical approach to breast disease. By presenting a way of thinking which clearly and thoroughly delineates the causes, the process, and the *connections* between and among breast disorders, it is my desire to give all women the means to minimize or avoid them altogether.

SECTION II

The Chinese Description & Treatment
Of Breast Diseases

CHAPTER I

Introduction

It should be obvious from the preceding discussion that the Chinese medical view of diseases of the breast is going to be very different from that of Western medicine. According to Chinese medicine, *all the diseases listed above are considered to be on one continuum and are not really separate at all.* In other words, premenstrual breast pain and distention is only the first stage of what may develop into other breast diseases such as breast lumps, whether painful or painless, or whether benign or malignant. This explains why women with what are considered by Western medicine to be benign breast diseases are more likely to develop breast cancer later in life. This progressive process is well delineated by traditional Chinese medicine. While using Western medical disease names, the chart below illustrates the Chinese medical idea of this continuum.

It is necessary to realize that this chart is only a possible visualization of the process of breast diseases. This continuum can

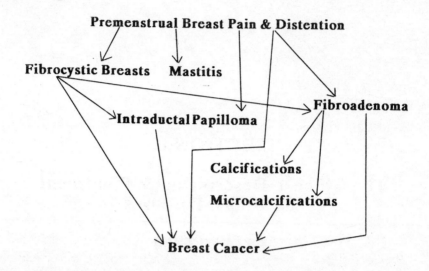

manifest with varying routes, *and successful intervention can take place at any point along those routes.* In order to understand how this continuum works, or how and why our bodies may follow one or another of these routes, it is necessary to explain some basic theories of Chinese medical physiology and pathology.

CHAPTER II

From Liver Qi To Lumps:
The Concept Of Stagnation

It is one thing to have some PMS symptoms with tender or swollen breasts each month for a few days. It is quite another to have carcinoma of the breast. The process of getting from the one to the other is complex, but according to Chinese medicine, *there is a very logical progression from distention to neoplasm.*

In order to understand this progression and also the specific breast disorders that Chinese medicine says make up the way stations along the route, one must understand the concept of Stagnation in Chinese medicine. This is a definite technical term within Chinese medicine (hence the capital letters) meaning any energy or substance in the body which is not flowing or being transformed properly. In Chinese medicine six things can become Stagnant in the body. These are Qi, Blood, Food, Dampness, Phlegm, and Fire. These Six Stagnations can, and, in fact, usually do arise in combination with one another. Initially, however, we will describe them separately.

Stagnant Qi

Qi (energy or lifeforce) can become Stagnant or Congested for a number of reasons. A traumatic injury can disrupt its flow, causing it to back up behind the injured area. Another of the Stagnations such as Blood, Food, or Dampness may impede its flow. However,

21

the *most* common cause of Qi Stagnation is a disturbance of what are called in Chinese medicine the Seven Emotions or Passions.

According to Chinese medical theory all emotions are nothing other than the subjective mental experience of the various manifestations of Qi. That is, the Qi and the Mind or emotions are not separate. The Qi of different Organs in the body will manifest emotionally in different ways, hence the Seven Emotions. (See Figure #6) Conversely, any externally induced emotional response can affect the Organ to which that emotion is related. An example of this phenomenon is having an upset or nervous stomach, perspiration, or movement of the bowels due to an emotional reaction to some external stimulus.

Figure 6.

THE SEVEN EMOTION ORGAN CORRESPONDANCES

HEART . . . . JOY/FRIGHT

SPLEEN . . . . WORRY

LUNG . . . . GRIEF/MELANCHOLY

KIDNEY . . . . FEAR

LIVER . . . . ANGER

However, it is especially those emotions related to stress, such as anger, frustration, worry, fear, vexation, and anxiety which will tend to Stagnate the Qi. Conversely, our experience of these emotions *is the experience of Stagnated Qi.*

To better understand this idea of emotions and their relationship to Organs, we must explain the concept of the Organs in Chinese Medicine.[20] Chinese medicine recognizes by name most of the same organs that we learn about in Western biology, but because

Chinese medicine is primarily energetic medicine, the definitions of Chinese Organs are largely energetic. The Chinese Organs are not just pieces of meat comprised of specific types of tissue, but rather functional orbs or zones of greatly concentrated energetic activity within the larger energetic grid or template of the body.[21] Each Organ is responsible for certain energetic functions which, in relationship to each other, keep the body healthy and in balance.

The balance and health of all the emotions is included in the energetic functions of the Organs. If an emotional response to an external stimulus arises, *and does not pass away in a natural and timely manner,* it can affect the Organ to which it is related. That is to say, emotions which are not resolved, but which affect a person for days, weeks, months, or longer, will usually impact upon the energy of the Organs in a deleterious manner. Thus we can see that without being able to test such things as galvanic skin response, temperature of the extremities, brain wave patterns, or other biofeedback measurements, the Chinese have known for millennia that mental/emotional activity strongly affects the activity of the internal viscera, and vice versa.

The Organ with which we are most concerned in relation to Stagnant Qi is the Liver. One of the major function of the Liver is to Promote Smoothing and Dispersal (of the Qi). The Liver is considered to be the tempermental Organ, that is, the one most affected by negative emotional disturbance or stress. If this happens, as it does endemically in our culture, the Liver quite commonly loses its ability to Smoothe and Disperse. That is merely a fancy way of saying that the Qi of the Liver loses its free flow and becomes Congested, or Stagnant.

There is a famous saying in Chinese medicine that goes "Where there is free flow, there is no pain; where there is pain, there is no free flow". Therefore, the main symptoms of the loss of free flow of the Qi in any part of the body is pain, and secondarily, distention. The pain will usually be of a crampy, diffuse nature. It may come and go, or vary in intensity at different times.

When Qi Stagnates in the Liver, or in any other Organ for that matter, it will also tend to Stagnate along the pathways over which that Qi travels, which we call the channels or meridians. Each Organ has one meridian to which it is most directly connected. The Liver meridian, also called in Chinese the Foot *Jue Yin* meridian, irrigates the lower abdomen and genitalia, the chest and flanks, the nipples, the throat, the gums, and the vertex of the head.

Earlier, I spoke of the the Organs being zones of greatly concentrated activity within the larger energetic grid or template of the body. The channels or meridians *are* the grid or template which circulate the energy of the Organs. You might think of them as the electromagnetic wiring of the body which allows movement, communication, and transformation between and among the Organs and tissues of the entire body. If the Qi in any Organ becomes stuck or Stagnant, symptoms of Stagnation may arise along the meridian or meridians most closely related to that Organ. This is *part* of the reason why Stagnant Liver Qi can lead to Stagnation in the breast tissue, evidenced by pain and distention. (See Figure #7 and #8)

Qi can Stagnate in Organs other than the Liver, but the Liver is the most common and usual place for Stagnant Qi to begin. As we will see later, however, if not dealt with in some healthy fashion, the Stagnation is not likely to stop there.

Stagnant Blood

Once again, there may be many causes for Stagnation of Blood. Like Qi Stagnation, it can be due to a traumatic injury damaging the vessels and causing the Blood to pool outside them, i.e. bruising, contusions, or hematomas. An insufficiency of either Qi or Blood can cause the Blood to Stagnate simply because there is just not enough Qi to move the Blood along, or not enough substance for it to be propelled. This is rather like a stream in autumn when some trickles of water are moving downstream, but some pockets of the water are just pooled in rocky areas and there is no longer enough flow to move them. The openings of the meridians and vessels then are not kept open by adequate flow of

24

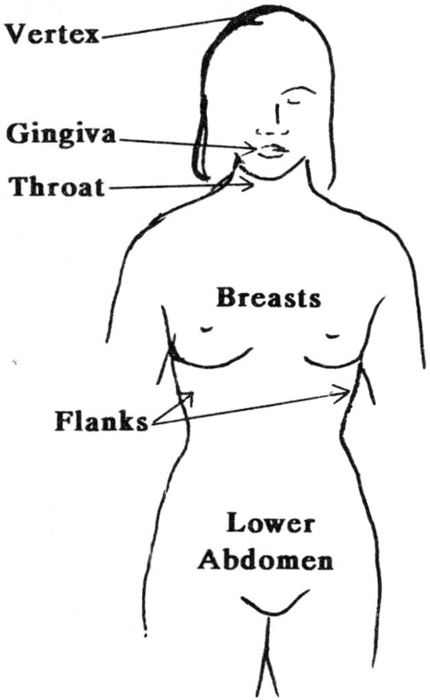

Pericardium (Hand *Jue Yin*) Meridian

Chong Mai - Penetrating Channel

Liver (Foot *Jue Yin*) Meridian

Stomach (Foot *Yang Ming*) Meridian

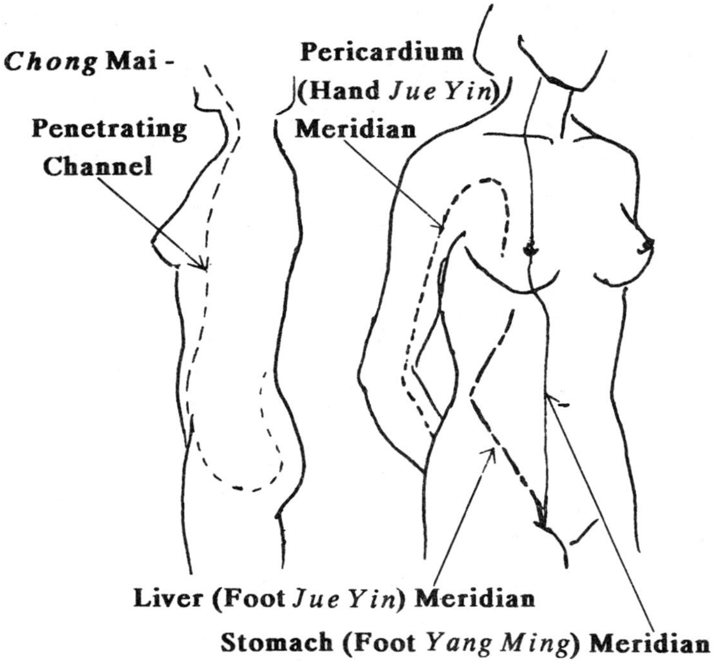

Figure 7. Meridian routes affecting the breast.

Vertex

Gingiva

Throat

Breasts

Flanks

Lower Abdomen

Figure 8. Liver Zones of Influence

Qi and Blood, and the Blood Stagnates. Also, it is one of the jobs of the Qi to move the Blood, so that if Qi becomes Deficient, it may not be strong enough to propel the Blood properly.

The third possibility is that Stagnant Qi may lead to Stagnant Blood. Because Qi and Blood flow together in the Channels and Vessels, if one becomes Stagnant, over time the other will also tend to become Stagnant.

In relation to Blood Stagnation the Liver again plays an important role. As mentioned in the section above, the Liver controls the Smoothing and Dispersal of Qi. Another function of the Liver is to Store the Blood, especially during times of inactivity such as sleep. Since it is the Qi which commands all movement of Blood, if the Liver Qi becomes Stagnant and remains so over a period of time, the Blood storing function of the Liver will also become impaired, and Blood movement irregular. Another way to say this is that the Blood stored by the Liver is moved by the Qi of the Liver; if the Liver Qi is Stagnant it cannot move the Blood in and out as required. Because the Liver (Foot *Jue Yin*) Channel flows through the uterus and genitalia, Stagnant Liver Qi which leads to Stagnant Blood will often manifest as some type of irregularity or difficulty with the menstrual flow. We will see later on how irregular menstruation relates to breast dysfunction.

There are other Organs which can be related to Stagnant Blood, especially the Heart and Stomach, but these will have less direct affect on breast disease than the scenario described above. Also, although Blood Stagnation is not usually one of the important factors in early stages of breast disease, it is an extremely important one in more serious types of breast disease. This indicates that if Blood Stagnation is longstanding it can have serious consequences, which in turn suggests that is it important to treat menstrual disorders which involve Blood Stagnation as early and as thoroughly as possible.

The signs of Blood Stagnation often include sharp, stabbing pain in a fixed area or spot, as in severe menstrual cramps. The tongue may be darkish or purple, possibly with dark patches or splotches.

26

There may be palpable lumps in the painful area, depending upon whether the Blood Stagnation is substantial or insubstantial. A practitioner of Chinese medicine might find the pulse at the radial artery to be deep and wiry or choppy. For more information about the possible diagnosis and treatment of Blood Stagnation related to the menses, I refer readers to *Free and Easy: Traditional Chinese Gynecology for American Women* by Bob Flaws, and especially the article "Premenstrual Syndrome: PMS".

Stagnant Food

This type of Stagnation can be very important in relation to breast diseases and should be well understood as it is one over which most of us have some control. Food Stagnation arises due to overeating. This can be a shortlived situation, as in feasting at holiday meals, or longterm, as in regular or constant overeating. The food then becomes Stagnant, which impedes the flow of Qi in the Stomach. If the Stomach Qi is impeded it cannot transport the food along its way properly, separating the Clear, or useable parts, from the Turbid, or unusable waste products, which further exacerbates the Food Stagnation. Also, since the nature of Qi in general is warm, if it is backed up behind Stagnant Food, or becomes Stagnant for any reason, it will tend to become Hot after some time. One symptom of a Hot Stomach is excessive appetite, encouraging the person to overeat even more. All this can become a vicious cycle.

If the Stomach is unable to combust food properly due to longterm Stagnation, the Stagnation becomes rather like sludge in a faulty carburator. This sludge will typically transform into Stagnant Phlegm, or Stagnant Phlegm Fire if it is not resolved in a healthy fashion. (See the section on Stagnant Phlegm below.)

Finally, Food Stagnation exacerbates any existing Qi Stagnation, especially any disharmonies between the Liver, Stomach, and Spleen. This complicating situation is so common that the representative guiding formula for activating Qi Stagnation, *Yue Ju Wan*, includes as one of its standard ingredients Massa Medica Fermentata, which is a famous food de-stagnating medicinal in

27

Chinese herbal medicine. That is also why it is recommended that people with Liver Qi Stagnation not overeat and limit hard to digest foods such as meat and nuts.

Stagnant Dampness

Dampness can be generated internally and invade the body from externally. Dampness may invade the body due to damp weather or working in a Damp environment. When this happens the movement of Qi can easily be obstructed, manifesting either as heaviness, stiffness, soreness in the joints, fullness in the chest or abdomen, or turbid, cloudy, or sticky secretions and excretions from the body. External Dampness may also affect the Spleen since is is said in the Chinese medical classics that "The Spleen fears Dampness."[22]

Disharmony of the Spleen may also generate Internal Dampness. It is the Spleen's job to transform Blood and Qi from the food and liquids sent to it by the Stomach. If the Spleen is dysfunctional or its Qi is Insufficient, it will be unable to transform liquids properly, thus leading to a condition of Internal Dampness. It is useful to note that Internal Dampness renders a person more susceptible to invasion of External Dampness and vice versa. Whether Internally or Externally generated, however, Dampness is heavy, turbid, and lingering, and by its nature tends to Stagnate, being difficult to remove from the body. Because this will tend to aggravate any existing Qi Stagnation, it can have a negative, if indirect effect on the breast. If not resolved it can be a precursor to the following type of Stagnation, which is a serious contributor to breast disorders.

Stagnant Phlegm

If Stagnant Dampness and Stagnant Food are left untreated, or linger for a long time, they may condense into Phlegm. In Chinese medicine this word has a much larger meaning than its connotations in Western medicine. Its generation is usually due to disharmony of the Spleen or Stomach, or both, as described in the two sections above. It is said in Chinese that "the Spleen is the Root of Phlegm".

This Phlegm may then:

1. lodge in the Lungs causing upper respiratory dysfunction;
2. obstruct the meridians where it may variously cause numbness, paralysis, lumps, nodules, or tumors;
3. obstruct the Heart where it disturbs the Spirit, causing behavioral changes, madness, or unconsciousness.

Phlegm is a common component of many types of neoplasms or lumps, whether benign or malignant, and is therefore an important element in breast diseases.

Stagnant Fire

I have stated above that Qi, or lifeforce, is by its nature warm. If enough Qi is trapped or Stagnated in one place for long enough time, the warmth can "ignite", transforming to Fire. Stagnant Fire, or body Heat that is not properly circulated and therefore combusts, is most typically found in the Liver due to longterm Stagnant Qi. This Fire may cause several types of symptoms. It may stay stuck in the Liver, causing the person to feel depressed, anxious, or irritable, but also to complain of cold extremities as the Heat is not circulated out to the rest of the body. There may also be pain in the ribs or flanks, and a bitter taste in the mouth upon waking in the morning.

Because the Liver itself is an Organ which does not like to hold on to Hot energies, the Stagnant Fire may be transferred to the Liver or Gallbladder meridians, (The Gallbladder is the Bowel paired with the Liver). In this scenario the Fire may rise, via these meridians, up to the head causing such symptoms as dizziness, red painful eyes, ringing in the ears, migraine headaches, insomnia, bleeding gums, or outbursts of inappropriate anger. It may also spread laterally to the Stomach, since the Liver and Stomach have

29

a strong Internal relationship, causing symptoms of Stomach Fire such as ravenous appetite, toothaches, sore breast tissue, or great thirst.

Stagnant Fire is usually seen as a strong pathogenic energy, one which is the end product of a fairly complex, lengthy process. It is difficult to remove and dissolve. Stagnant Fire is often a component of breast cancer.

Interrelationships

The above descriptions of the Six Stagnations are relatively brief and simple. However, they are a basic introduction to show how each one may be related to the breasts. It is also important to explain how these six energies may affect and interpromote each other. Below is a diagram of how these Stagnant energies may interrelate.

Figure 9.
Interrelationships of Stagnations

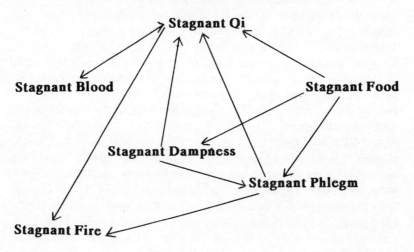

Because the Qi commands the Blood, unresolved Stagnant Qi can lead to Stagnant Blood. Because Qi is warm in nature, longterm Stagnant Qi can also lead to Stagnant Fire. Conversely, if the Blood Stagnates and remains unresolved it can impede the Qi flow, causing the Qi to Stagnate as well.

If the Spleen becomes weak, generating Dampness which lingers, the Dampness will both hinder the proper flow of Qi and hinder the Spleen's function of creating fresh Qi and Blood from the essence of the foods and liquids. If this happens the Qi and Blood may become weak or insufficient, and will also Stagnate for lack of sufficient amounts to propel themselves along. Additionally, if Stagnant Dampness lingers long enough, it can transform to Stagnant Phlegm which is much more difficult to remove.

Stagnant Food will also Stagnate the Qi and thus eventually lead to Stagnant Heat and Stagnant Blood.

Stagnant Phlegm will greatly hinder the normal flow of Qi wherever it is lodged. If Stagnant Qi transforms to Stagnant Fire, it will "stew" any Phlegm or Dampness with which it comes in contact. This can be described somewhat like the cooking of a dumpling. It starts out as a gooey, loosely formed mass, but the Fire solidifies it into a well-formed, hardened one. This is one of the major ways in which tumors are formed in the body.

If this process remains unchecked the ultimate finale is the production of what are called **Fire Toxins**. This term refers to Toxins formed by unresolved Stagnant Fire which has combined with Dampness and Phlegm and transformed into some type of supperative inflammation in the skin or other tissues. This type of Stagnancy is often seen in cases of carbuncles, boils, herpes lesions, and many types of cancer. **Damp Toxins** are similar in nature, except that they are produced by prolonged Stagnant Dampness, and they have a tendency to percolate downward in the body, as opposed to Heat or Fire, which has a tendency to rise.

These Six Stagnations will often be referred to in the following chapters, as they are major components in the process of all breast disease. In clinical practice it is important for the clinician to determine the varying proportions of each type of Stagnant energy or substance in order for proper treatment to take place.

CHAPTER III

The Worst Case Scenario

In the previous chapter the Six Stagnations were introduced, along with some of the Chinese Organs, the Chinese concept of Emotions, and the meridian system, with hints about how all this relates to the breast. Now let's try to make all this clearer, and fit the pieces together by way of a hypothetical example. This "case history" is a composite of several case histories illustrating a worst case scenario of the breast disease process or continuum. It is important to note that any individual situation may not proceed this way at all, and with proper intervention by a woman herself, and good Chinese medical care if symptoms do arise, *no woman's situation need develop in this way.*

Charlene, 27, is a recent graduate of law school and has landed a well paying but **stressful** position as an associate in a prestigious law firm. She has had a **history of minor diffuse menstrual cramps** on the first day of her period since menarche at 14. As her job becomes more complex and stressful, these **cramps worsen** and become occasionally stabbing, and she notices that she regularly has **sore, distended breasts** for four to seven days prior to her periods. She sometimes feels **irritable and depressed** at those times as well. All this precipitates a fight with her boyfriend, who feels she is spending too much time at work and that he is no longer a priority in her life. After two or three months

33

of these arguments, they break up and he moves out. She now must pay the full rent on their large and rather expensive apartment.

After several months of intermittent dating, she is **thoroughly frustrated** by the men she has met, the sexual pressure they place on her, along with her own sexual ambivalence and fear of disease. She spends more and more time working and avoids a social life altogether for some time. Due to her long hours and hard work, she is given more responsibility and higher pay at work, and the promise of a partnership in the firm at a later date.

Two years have passed and she is now almost 30. Her symptoms are the same, and she has sought no treatment for them other than taking an occasional tranquilizer to help her sleep when she gets **insomnia**, which happens once every few months. Now, however, she notices that, along with pain and distention, her breasts feel lumpy for the last week before her period. The lumpiness varies in amount and location from month to month, and the lumps disappear at the onset of menstruation. Her Western gynecologist tells her that she has **fibrocystic breast disease,** a benign condition for which there is no specific treatment unless she wishes to try progesterone therapy, or try going on birth control pills. He tells her to cut down on coffee, chocolate, and cola drinks and to see him if any lumps get worse or don't disappear with the onset of the period. Such lumps, he says, can be removed by aspiration in his office if they become too large or bothersome.

At age 31 she marries a fellow lawyer and her symptoms improve for about a year or so. She is working less during this period and feels more relaxed than she has since before law school. When she is 34, she decides that she would like to have a child before she gets any older. They have the money to afford a good full time nanny, and she will only have to take 3 months off after the pregnancy. Although it **takes her over a year to conceive** and she has three months of fairly severe **morning sickness,** she does carry the pregnancy to term. The labor drags on for several hours before her obstetrician suggests a **Caesarian section** due to lack of dilation of the cervix and indications of stress on the fetus.

34

After about one and one-half months of breast feeding, she develops **mastitis.** Her Western doctor gives her antibiotics to quell the infection, and another drug to dry up her milk since she will no longer be able to nurse her baby. This being the case, she decides to return to full time work earlier than she had originally intended.

At age 36 she is made full partner in her law firm; consequently the **stress level in her life is higher.** Juggling her work and her responsibilities as a mother and wife are taking their toll. Her symptoms begin to worsen again, and this time one painful lump in her breast no longer disappears with the onset of menstruation. Her gynecologist diagnoses a **fibroadenoma** and suggests surgical removal if it has not decreased in size within six months. This is done, but it does not change her symptoms which now include **excessive appetite** with no weight gain, **cravings for sweets** before the period, with **occasional diarrhea and fatigue,** especially when her schedule is too hectic, or if she and her husband have a fight.

Charlene and her husband are divorced when she is 39 and their child is 5 years old. Now she must add the stress of single parenting and visitation schedules to her already stretched calendar. Her **periods become irregular** and more painful, with stabbing pain on the first day and diffuse cramps for several more days. The breasts continue to be lumpy, but she has gotten used to the cycle, and just takes a strong pain reliever when things get bad, or a tranquilizer when she gets too **irritable or anxious.** She is too busy to try and change her situation, and she has never thought of looking into any alternative approaches. Her doctor has suggested only that if the periods are too painful she might consider having a hysterectomy.

During a regular check-up with her MD he suggests that since she is now 41 she should have a base line mammogram done, continuing to get one every year since she has a history of fibrocystic disease. Her third mammogram at age 43 reveals a small, non-palpable lump that does not conform to the pattern of the other fibrocystic lumps. This **lump is biopsied and found to**

35

be cancerous, though it has apparently not spread to the lymph nodes in the surrounding area. A simple lumpectomy is performed, followed by a few sessions of radiation therapy. At that point, since no further cancer is found, she is told to come in for regular follow-up exams, but receives no more treatment.

During the later stages of menopause at age 50 Charlene notices that the same breast that had the malignancy removed is **occasionally weeping from the nipple.** The discharge is clear or slightly pinkish at first, but after a few weeks it becomes thicker and more brownish or yellow. **A Stage II Carcinoma in situ** is discovered with lymph node involvement this time. A radical mastectomy must be performed to remove all the affected tissue. Charlene has a 50/50 chance of surviving five years.

A sad, but not improbable tale.

Let's go back to the beginning and explain the entire process of Charlene's case, one symptom at a time, in terms of Chinese medical theory.

1. Diffuse menstrual cramps starting at menarche. Diffuse menstrual cramps are a common symptom of Liver Qi Stagnation. As we explained earlier, the Liver Channel irrigates the genitalia and the lower abdomen. One of the most common areas of the body to manifest Liver Qi Stagnation, especially in women, is the pelvis. The Qi commands the movement of the Blood. If the Qi is Stagnant, the Blood will have a difficult time flowing down and out freely. The Qi impeding the menstrual blood's free flow is experienced as cramping.

2. The cramps worsen with the higher stress level, becoming occasionally stabbing. At this point the Stagnant Liver Qi is not just impeding the flow of the menstrual blood, but it begins to cause the Blood to become Stagnant in the pelvis in a more serious way. The cramps then go from minor and diffuse in nature to sharp and stabbing. In fact, most women's cramps are some combination of both, showing that both the Qi and the Blood are Stagnant in varying proportions.

36

3. Depression and irritability. To explain the depression and irritability we must return to our discussion of the functions of the Liver. Along with storing the Blood and Smoothing and Dispersing the Qi, "the Liver stores or treasures the *Hun*".[23] The *Hun* is the Chinese word for our concept of the psyche, ego, or personality. If the Liver Qi is Stuck, the emotional corollary of that stuckness will be depression, frustration, or pent up anger. Anger and irritability is nothing other than rising Liver Qi. Depression is nothing other than stuck or Stagnated Liver Qi (anger which cannot rise). Both anger and depression are common symptoms of a Liver Qi disorder.

4. Painful, distended breasts. It is at this point in Charlene's story that we have the addition of sore and distended breasts prior to the period. To account for this symptom we must return to Figure 7 on page 27 showing the meridians which affect the breast tissue. This illustrations shows that the Liver (Foot *Jue Yin*) meridian, Pericardium (Hand *Jue Yin*), and Stomach (Foot *Yang Ming*) meridian are the most important in relation to the breast. First, let's discuss the Pericardium and Liver meridians. You will notice they have the same Chinese name, one being the hand, the other being the foot. This is because they share the same energetic level according to traditional Chinese physiology. The Pericardium meridian is sometimes seen as an extension of the Liver meridian in the upper body.[24] If the Qi in the Liver (Foot *Jue Yin*) meridian becomes Stagnant, it will tend to Stagnate the Pericardium (Hand *Jue Yin*) meridian as well because of this connection. Since we know that the Liver is the "tempermental" Organ, high stress jobs or lifestyles will tend to show their effects first on the Liver or its sphere of influence. This includes the *Jue Yin* meridians, both of which irrigate the breast tissue.

As we discussed in the chapter on the Six Stagnation, the Liver and the Stomach have a strong internal relationship. If the Liver becomes congested and therefore overheated, the Stomach may participate in this Heat and Congestion, causing the smooth flow of Qi over the Stomach (Foot *Yang Ming*) meridian to be impeded. The Stomach meridian directly irrigates the breast tissue. If the Qi or energy in this meridian is not flowing freely,

37

pain and distention of the breast tissue will be a common symptom.

Dr. Zhu Xiao-nan further describes these relationships:

> (Dr) Zhu says that the primary factor in this condition (breast pain and distention) is Liver Qi Congestion. Due to emotional excess, anger, frustration, and stress, the Liver Qi loses its free-flowing patency. This results in Excess Qi in the Liver which vents on or invades the Stomach... Therefore, there is simultaneous disturbance, i.e. congestion, in both the Foot *Jue Yin* (Liver channel) and the Foot *Yang Ming* (Stomach channel) meridians. Nipple pain (Liver) and breast distention (Stomach) are examples of this mutual involvement between these two Organs. Zhu emphasizes this close connection between stuck and knotted Liver Qi and breast distention. He recounts a story of a woman who had premenstrual breast distention. Once, during mid-cycle when her breasts were otherwise not sore or distended, she became very angry and upset. Immediately her breasts swelled up and became sore just as if she were premenstrual. This is Zhu's way of stressing the importance of psychoemotional factors in this disorder.[25]

5. Occasional insomnia. In number three above we mentioned that the Liver treasures the *Hun*, or psyche. It is the Liver's Blood storing function that allows the *Hun* to "rest" in the Liver. If the Liver Qi is Stagnant over a long enough time to Transform to Fire, it can waste, dry, or agitate the Blood making it unable to store the *Hun* properly.

This same Fire may also transfer to the Heart, agitating or wasting the Heart Blood. The Heart, as we said earlier, treasures the *Shen* or Spirit. If the Heart Blood is weakened or agitated, the *Shen* will become uneasy, not calm. Either of these two situations often lead to insomnia or dream disturbed sleep.

38

6. The breasts become lumpy before the period. The appearance of lumps which come and go, fibrocystic disease, are not different from the scenario described above in number four, they are just a further development of the Stagnant Qi. In Chinese medicine this condition, and fibroadenoma as well, come under the category of *Ru-Pi* (Breast Obstruction). In the *Yong Yi Da Quan* by Gu Shi it states

> "*Ru-Pi* is a nodule (or nodules) that appears on the breast. Its shape is like an egg or pellet. There may be a painful or heavy sensation, though pain may be absent. The surrounding skin is unchanged in color. The lump varies in size according to the mood of the woman..."[26]

As the Qi Stagnates, moves more freely, then Stagnates again, the lumps or nodules will appear and disappear. In *Acupuncture Case Histories From China,* edited by Chen and Wang it states

> "...breast masses are attributed primarily to emotional disturbance, which leads to stagnation of Liver Qi. Stagnation of Qi and stasis of Blood then develop into masses."[27]

At this point it is appropriate to explain how and why the menstrual cycle affects the energy circulating in the breasts, and why they tend to be most aggravated during the premenstrual week.

Week one: At the onset of the period the Blood in the uterus is full to overflowing. This Blood is moved down and out by the Qi.

Week Two: At this point after the period is over the Blood is relatively Deficient. Since it takes Blood to enfold and keep the Qi down, if the Blood is insufficient, the Qi, being warm in nature, will rise like a hot air balloon (Qi) from which the ballast (Blood) has been ejected. Therefore, the Qi rises towards the upper part of the body.

Week Three: At midcycle the Blood has become full again. The

39

Qi reaches its peak and now begins to move down.

Week Four: Now the Qi is trying to descend into the lower half of the body in order to move the Blood down and out. At the same time the Blood is full to Excess. Although in some women symptoms may appear with ovulation at midcycle, it is during this fourth week that *most* women who are affected by this problem will experience distended, painful, or lumpy breasts. If the Liver Qi is Stagnant, the Qi will not move freely into the pelvis. Instead it will get stuck as it tries to descend, causing distention and pain in the lower abdomen (premenstrual bloating), and/or in the breasts.

In relationship to the menses and the breasts there are two other meridians which play a crucial role. These are called the *Chong* and *Ren* meridians. They are two of what are called the Eight Extraordinary Meridians. The *Ren* meridian controls the functions of the uterus. The *Chong* meridian shares the same name as the uterus itself, the Sea of Blood, and is directly connected to it. The Qi of the *Ren* meridian, along with the Qi of the Liver, is responsible for moving the Blood in the *Chong* meridian and the uterus. Also, the *Chong* and *Ren* meridians connect with the Liver and the Stomach meridians in the lower abdomen at several points. This connection is clinically quite important -- so much so that it is said in Chinese, *Gan Ju Xue Hai*, or "Liver Controls the Sea of Blood". Therefore, if the Liver Qi is Stagnant, it may cause disharmony between and among any or all of the related meridians, leading to irregular menstruation as well as breast disease.

This is succinctly stated by Dr. Al Khafaji as follows:

> Although a number of channels traverse the breasts, it is the Stomach channel and the *Chong Mai* that supply and nourish them. A disorder of either of these channels can give rise to pathology of the breast.

> In almost all cases of *Ru-pi*, stagnation plays a crucial

part, whether it be via the Stomach channel (usually in the earlier stages) or via the *Chong Mai* (in the later stages).[28]

and by Dr. Zhu Xiao-nan:

> The Liver meridian traverses the reproductive organs. Problems in the reproductive organs are often related to or caused by Liver disharmony...When the menses is just about due, the Sea of Blood (uterus) is full and there may be tenderness in the hypogastrium. Therefore, if there is Liver Qi Congestion, it will be aggravated and consequently will display clear symptoms at this time. Above there will be chest oppression and breast distention and below there will be hypogastric pain and distention.

> After the menstrual flow begins, the Sea of Blood gradually empties. Therefore, the tender feeling diminishes. The Liver Stagnation softens and harmonizes and the breast and abdominal distention are leveled. This cycle repeats itself over and over again.[29]

7. Improvement in symptoms with a new marriage. It is interesting to note that a new and happy love relationship brought about a general improvement in Charlene's symptoms. This underscores the emotional nature of so many gynecological diseases. When a woman is within the comfort and support of a happy relationship, she relaxes more and her symptoms are somewhat alleviated. Additionally, a healthy and fulfilling sex life helps to circulate the Qi in the pelvis and thereby in the meridians which affect the breast tissue as well.

8. Difficulty conceiving. According to Chinese medicine the key to infertility in most women is the regularity of their menstrual cycle. If the menstruation is adjusted normally, there should be no problem conceiving. Irregular menses is *most* often at least partially, if not solely, due to Liver Qi Congestion, there being the connection between irregular menses and diseases of the breasts.

41

It is interesting to note that in China, most women with premenstrual breast distention, pain, or lumps *initiate* traditional herbal or acupuncture therapy not for the breast problem itself, but for infertility.[30] In records of 20 Chinese women with breast distention, all of them had difficulty conceiving.[31]

9. Morning sickness. This common condition can have many causes, but in the case we are presenting the main reason is similar to the situation just prior to menstruation. During pregnancy the discharge from the Sea of Blood does not occur and the lower part of the body is full. If the woman has any tendency towards Liver Qi Congestion, the Liver Qi cannot circulate into the lower body and may accumulate to the point where it vents across the Middle Burner and invades the Stomach. The Stomach's normal functioning is impinged upon by the Liver Qi and the Stomach Qi then rises along with the Liver Qi, in opposition to its regular direction or descension.

10. Difficult labor with Caesarian section. Women with Liver Qi Stagnation are prime candidates for painful labors. It is the Liver Qi and the Qi in the *Ren* channel which are responsible for discharging the menstrual Blood from the uterus and discharging the fetus from the uterus through labor. If the Qi is Stagnant, the movement will be difficult and there will be pain. Most Western obstetricians will respond to this pain with various types of drug therapy to eliminate the pain, or by Caesarian section if the labor lasts so long as to endanger the baby's life.

Because any meridians flowing through the region are severed, a Caesarian section cuts the meridians, disrupting the normal flow of Qi in the lower abdomen, in time increasing any existing Stagnation. The meridians affected include the Liver, Stomach, Kidney, *Chong* and *Ren*, three of which will directly affect the breasts.

11. Mastitis. This is a common complaint among women breast-feeding a first child. It is an inflammation of the breast characterized by pain, distention, redness and swelling, with blocked lactation, and often cold or flu-like symptoms such as

42

aversion to wind or chill, headache, and fever, or nausea.[32] In Chinese medicine mastitis is called *Ru Yong*, breast abscess, and is considered to be caused by either Liver Qi Congestion alone or in combination with the invasion of an External pathogen and overindulgence in fatty or rich foods which overheat and congest the Stomach and Liver. This pathogen obstructs the flow of Qi and Blood, especially in the Foot *Yang Ming* Stomach meridian which irrigates the breast. The obstruction causes retention of milk. The retention of milk and the toxic Heat collect in the breast, causing pain, redness, and swelling. There also may be systemic fever, thirst, constipation, and nausea. This is often complicated by a background of Liver Qi Congestion related to post-partum depression, anxiety, or feelings of being overwhelmed, all of which are common in new mothers. Such feelings, or any type of stress, will exacerbate any tendency of the Liver to become Hot. This Liver Heat will then participate with any pathogen invading from the outside, thereby complicating the diagnosis and treatment. This would suggest that women with prior breast complaints due to Liver Qi Congestion may be more susceptible to mastitis.

12. Fibroadenoma. At this point in Charlene's story we must return to Stagnation of Phlegm. We have shown how Qi Stagnation will cause a disharmony between the Liver and the Stomach. If this continues over time the disharmony will extend to include the Spleen. This is because the Spleen and Stomach work together as an pair, and any influence on one will often influence the other. One of the Spleen's jobs is to move and transform liquids. If this function of the Spleen is compromised due to an imbalance with the Liver energy, or for any other reason, Dampness will collect and Phlegm will be generated. If the Liver and Stomach are also Hot, this Phlegm will be drafted up like creosote or soot is drafted up a chimney. It may deposit in the breasts (or neck, or underarm area) and "stewed" like the dumpling we mentioned earlier, hardening into nodules. These nodules may still fluctuate in size with the mood of the woman, but they will no longer disappear altogether. These nodules are what Western medicine calls severe fibrocystic lumps or fibroadenomas. In Chinese medicine these are called *Ru-Pi*, Breast Obstruction.

43

13. Craving for sweets; excess appetite; occasional diarrhea and fatigue. This set of symptoms confirms our discussion of Stomach Heat and Spleen weakness in #12 above (fibroadenomas). When the Stomach becomes Hot there will be increased appetite but usually no weight gain, as if the Stomach were working overtime like an engine in which the idle speed is turned up too high. The diarrhea and craving for sweets go together and are related to the Spleen. The Spleen must separate the most refined part of the food and liquids we ingest into the Pure and the Impure parts, sending the Pure up and the Impure down, transforming liquids and creating Qi and Blood in this process. If the Spleen is disorded by the "invasion" of Stagnant Liver Qi it can become weakened and unable to perform these jobs. The Pure and Impure are not completely separated, liquids not properly transformed, leading to diarrhea.

Craving sweets relates to the concept of the Five Flavors. Each major Organ has one flavor to which it most "attracted" or related. Because Sweet is the flavor most associated with the Spleen, when the Spleen is weak it may crave its related flavor, even though large amounts of the Sweet flavor will further weaken it.

If the Spleen is not able to create proper amounts of Qi and Blood due to weakness, there will be fatigue, which is one of the most common signs of Spleen Qi Deficiency.

14. Irregular Periods with Stabbing Cramps. Irregular menstruation in American women is usually caused by Stagnation, either of Qi, Blood, Fire, or a combination of these. In this scenario we have a combination of Stagnant Qi which has continued for some years, leading to Stagnant Blood.

We have said that Stagnation gives rise to pain. The pain of Stagnant Qi will be relatively diffuse, possibly moving from place to place and varying in intensity. Pain that is fixed and stabbing, however, indicates Stagnant Blood. While the Stagnant Blood may not affect the breasts directly at first, it is in this case an indication that longterm Qi Stagnation exacerbated by lower abdominal surgery has taken its toll on the body's normal circulation of energy

44

and Blood in the pelvis and the meridians which irrigate it.

In our earlier discussion of breast pain (see #6 above) we spoke about the channels which traverse and nourish the breast, namely the Foot *Yang Ming* (Stomach), the Foot *Jue Yin* (Liver), and the *Chong Mai*. We also said that the *Chong* and *Ren* channels control menstruation. The *Chong* and the uterus share the same name, the Sea of Blood. If the Blood is Stagnant in the uterus, causing stabbing cramps, it will eventually also be Stagnant in the *Chong Mai*. This channel is like the internal polar axis of the body and is the deepest layer of our energetic being. It nourishes the breast at a very deep level, while the Stomach channel nourishes the breast at a more superficial level. If there is Stagnant Blood in the *Chong Mai* channel it will eventually affect the breasts at this deep level. In fact, while the earlier stages of breast diseases are more often directly related to the Stomach and Liver and their meridians, most later stages of breast disease are related to Stagnation in the *Chong Mai*.

Before going on to discuss Charlene's final devolution into cancer, let us sum up her hypothetical history to emphasize the most important points. She has experienced the full continuum of breast disease, beginning with Stagnation of Liver Qi giving rise to breast pain and other PMS symptomology. The most important things to note overall in her story are:

> 1. That she passed each warning signpost without adequate treatment, and,
>
> 2. That she did nothing to reduce or control the stress in her life.

By the time we get to age 43 and the lumpectomy, this process is much more difficult to abort than it would have been 15, 10, or even 5 years earlier. *The single most important key to stopping this process at any stage along the way has mostly to do with dealing effectively with emotional stress.* This not having been done in Charlene's case, the cancer was not an unlikely finale to her health difficulties. Let us now take a look at the Chinese description of breast cancer. Because it is such an important and extensive subject, it will be discussed in a chapter by itself.

CHAPTER IV

The Chinese Medical View
Of Breast Cancer

In Chinese medicine breast cancer has several names. It can be called *Du Ru*, Breast Obstruction, *Gou Chao Ru*, Breast Fistula, *Ru Tong Jian*, Pain and Firmness of Breast, *Ru Shi Tong Nai Yan*, Painful Breast as Hard as a Rock, or *Ru Yan*, Breast Rock.[33] It is described as being caused by none other than the things which have been discussed in this book already. This will include Stagnation of Liver Qi due to emotional stress, Spleen Dampness, Stagnant Blood, Stagnant Phlegm, Heat, and Toxins, usually in some combination and having lasted for many years.[34] Several quotations will further illustrate these points.

In *The Orthodox Manual of External Disease* of the Ming dynasty it is pointed out that:

> Breast cancer is due to worry and melancholy. Lots of ideas hanging around make one feel dissatisfied. Perverse flow of Liver *Qi* to the Spleen leads to the Obstruction of the Channels....[35]

From *Carcinoma* by Jia Kun,

> Breast cancer is mainly caused by the disturbed

emotions such as grief, bitter weeping, fear, worry and depression, or by improper sexual life without paying attention to hygiene, or by increased excretion of estrogen. It is also closely related to artificial abortion, early terminated pregnancy, single life, no breast feeding and improper breast feeding. After menopause, the deteriorated function of the nervous system, the impaired excretion of ovarian hormone, the blocked regulation of the ovaries by nervous system and some other diseases can also result in breast cancer.[36]

And finally, from *Treating Cancer with Chinese Herbs* by H.Y. Hsu,

...breast cancer is linked to the seven passions and exhaustion of blood in the liver meridian, the melancholic accumulation of liver vitality, and obstruction of *ch'i* (Qi). Also, coagulation of blood caused by irregular menses can turn into a hard mass...[37]

A very specific breakdown of the causes of breast cancer is given in *The Treatment of Cancer by Integrated Chinese-Western Medicine,* by Zhang Dai-zhao as follows:

1. Qi Stagnation due to Liver Depression
2. Phlegm Dampness due to Spleen Deficiency
3. Stagnant Toxins
4. Deficiency of Both Qi and Blood [38]

We have discussed all of these with the exception of number four in some detail in various preceeding sections . The material presented so far indicates that the *major* cause of breast diseases is usually some combination of two or more of the Six Stagnations. A Stagnation is by its nature a form of Excess, so how can Deficiency of Qi and Blood relate to these Stagnations?

48

The free and patent flow of Qi and Blood are dependent upon there being enough of each of them for propulsion. In the section on Blood Stagnation in Section II, Chapter II, the analogy of a stream in autumn was given to describe Blood Deficiency. This is when there is just not a large enough volume of Blood to keep the channels open and the Blood moving, thereby leading to Blood Stagnation.

The mechanism of Qi Deficiency is slightly different. One of the jobs of the Qi is to move the Blood. When there is too little Qi the Blood will not move properly, thereby causing it to become Stagnant over time.

Another job of the Qi is to hold the Blood and Fluids within their proper vessels or tissues. When the Qi is Deficient, there may arise symptoms of bleeding or leakage of fluid from any of the body orifices. In Charlene's case, one of her symptoms in the second appearance of breast cancer is galactorrhea, a discharge from the nipple. At first the discharge is clear, indicating Qi Deficiency, with some blood, also indicating the presence of Pathogenic Heat. After a week or two, the discharge becomes turbid and dark. This shows that the cancerous lesions in her breast are not only Hot, but also Toxic in nature.

RISK FACTORS

Certain factors are said by Western medical sources to increase a woman's chances of breast cancer. These usually can be explained locically by Chinese medical theory.

1. Aging: One possible explanation for the increased incidence in breast cancer in women over 40 is that as a woman becomes older the Fluids and Blood (Yin) in her body become Deficient in relationship to the Heat and Qi (Yang). This is the natural process of aging, where the body tissues are not able to be nourished by the diminishing Blood and Fluids, so that they become dry and withered. This same process that is being reflected on the Outside is happening on the Inside as well. This slowly progressing

49

imbalance of Yang and Yin, Qi and Blood, which is part of the normal process of aging, allows any Stagnant Qi that may be in the body to be more easily transformed into Stagnant Fire because there is less Blood and Fluid available to moisten dryness and keep Qi and Heat (Yang) in check, or enfolded.

Additionally, after menopause, a woman can no longer discharge Heat and Toxicity from her body each month via the menstruation. This allows for a more pronounced build up of any pathogenic energies which may be present in the body. Furthermore, as we age, our production of Qi and Blood decreases, making Stagnation due to Qi and Blood Deficiency all the more likely.

Finally, any one of the Six Stagnations, or even a combination of two or three, will not often become so Hot or so Toxic in a short time as to cause cancer to develop. *Most often* it takes some years for any disease process to become so life-threatening.

2. Early Menarche (onset of menstruation): It is also said that women who experienced an early menarche have a slightly higher risk of breast cancer. One of the first signs of menarche is the budding of the breasts. The breast tissue is irrigated and controlled by the Liver and Stomach energy. This budding, if it happens early, shows a tendency for the Qi in these channels to already be somewhat Excess, even at such a young age.

3. Family history: Chinese medicine is not very clear in its descriptions of what diseases or disease tendencies may be inherited. It is my personal opinion however, that this influence must be put largely in the category of learned behavior. We have all learned from our parents, grandparents, and other family members, how to cope with life and its various stresses. Because cancer is a disease that is often closely related to the emotions, it is difficult to substantiate an *inherited tendency* to produce the same disease as one's mother or sister in the case of cancer. I feel that it is more likely one has learned to respond to life's various challenges and stresses in the same ways as did her mother and sister. It is also possible for members of the same family to be affected by the same environmental or dietary carcinogens.

50

4. Overweight and a high fat diet: A woman's diet, and her relationship to regular exercise are at least to some extent, learned behaviors. Statistics from the National Institute of Childhood Health and Human Development show that people whose parents are overweight have a much higher than average chance of also being overweight, and that this tendency is not genetic as much as it is learned behavior.[39]

High fat or greasy foods are considered in Chinese medicine to produce Dampness and Phlegm. As we have explained previously, these substances will have a tendency to Stagnate the Qi, transform into Heat or Hot Phlegm, and if present in the body for a long enough time, become lumps or nodulations, i.e. tumors either benign or malignant.

5. History of benign breast diseases: As was stated in the introduction to this book, Chinese medicine sees the occurrence of any breast disease as related to the occurrence of other breast disease, not as discrete pathologies. Cancer is merely considered to be a breast disease that has been present in some form for long enough to become extremely virulent. Its diagnostic parameters are not *fundamentally* different from benign breast diseases. It is only logical then that a history of benign breast disease would predispose a woman to a higher risk for breast cancer.

6. Late or no childbearing: In Chinese medicine giving birth is energetically similar to having a period. In both cases, something collects in the uterus over a period of time and then is discharged. During the period, it is Blood which is discharged. During labor it is a baby. Although the end product is quite dissimilar, the process is much the same. In both instances the body opens up in order to let something out. In Chinese medicine, the menstrual discharge is considered a somewhat Turbid substance. It is not entirely Pure. If this Turbid Blood is not discharged completely, it will lead to the accumulation of Stagnant Blood, Turbidity, and Heat in the pelvic region. Likewise, besides resulting in a newborn child, parturition also results in a very large discharge of Turbid Blood. Such a discharge is very cleansing and potentially healing. Women who delay childbirth or choose not to have children biologically either

51

delay or deny this large cleansing and opening discharge. Therefore, any tendency towards Stagnation of Qi and Blood will continue to build rather than being swept away with labor and the post-partum lochia (blood discharge). (This is why many women's menstrual complaints spontaneously improve or disappear with childbirth.) If this Stagnation in the pelvis, and therefore the Liver, is allowed to continue building, this may eventually cause Stagnation and Accumulation in the breasts due to the internal connections of the Liver and Stomach and their meridians.

7. Late menopause: The *Nei Jing*, the first classic of Chinese medicine, states that in women menopause should occur at around 49 years of age. The menstrual discharge is not exactly Pure Blood but it is Blood in any case. Blood is created out of the Essence of the of Food and Liquids in the Spleen and the Congenital Essence stored in the Kidneys.[39] Since, in Chinese medicine, the Kidneys are responsible for the aging process, the healthier the Kidneys are, the slower the person will age. Because of the decline in Blood production in turn due to the natural decline in digestion after age 35, monthly loss of the menstruate after that has a tendency to weaken the Kidneys. When the body recognizes this through its own homeostatic wisdom, it shuts down menstruation so as to prevent further loss of Kidney Essence through this discharge. After menopause, since Blood is not being discharged on a monthly basis, the Kidney Essence is consumed much more slowly and the woman can go on to live another 30 years in relative good healthy and with slow, gradual aging.

In Chinese medicine, women who experience a later than normal cessation of menstruation may do so because of any of three reasons. First, they may have such strong Kidney Essence and such good digestion that they continue producing a superabundance of Blood longer than most other women. Although these women experience menopause relatively late, they tend, however, to be healthier than the average. Secondly, some women are Hotter internally than others. Usually this Excess Heat or Excess Yang arises and manifests in the Liver and Stomach. In Chinese medicine it is said that Heat makes the Blood run recklessly outside its pathways. In terms of menstruation, this most often causes

52

metrorrhagia (bleeding between periods), early periods, and menorrhagia (excessively heavy bleeding during the periods). However, this Heat can also force the Blood out of the uterus past when such discharge is, in fact, a healthy occurrence. Because of the connection between the Liver and Stomach, as the source of this Heat, and the breasts, this scenario can also commonly cause an accumulation of Heat and Stagnation in the mammary tissue.

The third Chinese medical reason for late menopause is that the woman's Qi is not strong enough to hold the Blood within the uterus. Therefore, the Blood tends to "fall" out inappropriately. This will, over time, also lead to Blood Deficiency since a 50 year old woman's Blood production is not sufficient to replace this lost Blood every 28 days. Often these women develop a continuous trickle of dysfunctional uterine bleeding. Since, as mentioned above, Deficiency of Qi and Blood can also cause breast disease, women with this type of delayed menstruation are also more prone to mastoses. Furthermore, since the Blood is Yin and the Woman's Yin is getting weak or is being relatively exhausted at this point in her life anyway, her Yang is tending to flare and cause Heat. Therefore, it is not uncommon for a woman to be both Qi and Blood Deficient and to also be over-heated as well. When these two conditions combine, they are even more likely to cause breast disease.

CONCLUSION

The most important lesson to learn from Charlene's "case history" and this discussion of cancer is that this continuum need not have proceeded to its unfortunate conclusion. Because Chinese medicine can describe the disease mechanisms at work in the case of each symptom, it can also treat and potentially prevent the symptoms as well, thus aborting the process before it becomes life-threatening. The following chapters in Section III discuss the prevention and treatment of breast diseases.

First, however, I'd like to describe the disease names and patterns of disharmony which Chinese medicine uses to break down this continuum of disease into comprehensible and treatable parts.

CHAPTER V

Chinese Categories Of Breast Disease

In Chinese medicine there are two parts to the diagnosis of any disorder. First is the disease category or name *(Bing)*, and second is the pattern or description of the cause *(Zheng)*. It is customary to discriminate the disease category first, and then discriminate what pattern or combination of patterns are responsible for that disease.

The *Essentials of Conformation in Chinese Medicine* and *Terminology of Chinese Medicine* list seven classical categories *(Bing)* of breast diseases[40], as follows:

1. Breast abscess or carbuncle (*Ru Yong*). This is another name for mammitis or mastitis. It is considered to be an Obstruction of the milk due to Invasion of an External pathogen, or due to injury from Internally generated Heat. There may be redness, swelling or hardness, and pain, obstructed milk flow, systemic fever, and a discharge from the nipple of milk or pus.

2. Breast ulcers (*Ru Zhu*). This is similar to #1 except that the ulcers form deep inside the breast and may cause a suppurating lesion on the surface of the breast. It is due to melancholy (excessive emotions) leading to accumulation of Excess Liver Qi and Heat in the Stomach causing a high fever. The surface of the lesion will weep yellow pus and may leave a deep hole in the skin.

3. Breast ulcers (*Ru Gan*). These ulcers erupt on the nipple or the areola. They characteristically develop on cracked or infected skin caused by nursing with improper hygiene. They are believed to be caused by Damp and Hot Toxins as were described above in the section on the Six Stagnations, complicated by the Stagnation of Blood and Qi. The condition is quite painful, and there is a mucous discharge from the nipple. This can easily transform into condition #1.

4. Breast swelling (*Ru Li*). The swelling resembles a grape. It is located in the middle of areola, and there is mild pain but the lump does not burst. After several months, it may naturally and suddenly dissipate. It is said to be due to Qi Obstruction and Phlegm Accumulation.

5. Chronic breast swelling (*Ru Pi*). This swelling takes the form of a movable, egg-shaped lump in the breast. It develops from Internal Injury by the Seven Passions harming the Liver and Spleen, Qi Obstruction, and Phlegm Stagnation. The lump tends to expand and contract with the woman's emotional state and mood. There is generally no pain, no change in skin color, and no bursting of the flesh.

6. Breasts consumption (*Ru Lao*). This condition, like #5 above, is caused by Qi Obstruction and Phlegm Stagnation. Its name suggests that chronic fatigue play a parat in it development. First, a hard mass the size of a small plum, that moves when palpated, is found. The center of the mass will be harder than the edges. If not treated, this condition will become painful and may burst internally, spreading Hot Toxins into the chest and ribs. At this stage it will be difficult to treat, and healing will be slow.

7. Galactorrhea or breast leakage (*Ru Lou*). This situation arises if there has been one of the above conditions and it has remained untreated, causing the body to become generally weak. The discharge may be either clear or odorous and may ooze for

56

months after treatment.

Within each of these disease categories, any one of several patterns of disharmony *(Zheng)* may be the root cause, or parts of one combine with parts of another. How they combine will depend upon a woman's underlying constitution and predispositions, and the balance between and among the various Organs. Presented below are the most common of the patterns seen in breast disease, listed on a continuum based upon complexity and seriousness. For each pattern the signs and symptoms as well as the disease mechanisms will be explained. This information is partially excerpted from the articles by Dr. Zhu Xiao-nan, translated and with commentary by Bob Flaws[41], and Mazin Al-Khfaji[42], both referred to above. The material presented here is similar to what is covered in the hypothetical case history description of symptoms above, but from a more clinically oriented viewpoint.

1. Stagnation of Liver Qi

This pattern forms the basis of all the other patterns of breast pain and distention *(RuPi)*. It is mostly seen in younger women, or in the first stages of the disorder.

Signs and Symptoms: Suppressed and depressed emotions; long-term anger and frustration are common; distention and pain of the breasts, chest, and flank; the pain may radiate to the back and shoulders; much sighing; Plum-seed Qi[43] in the throat, dream-disturbed sleep; irregularity of the menstrual cycle; irritability; tendency to constipation; pain and distention of the lower abdomen just prior to menstruation; all symptoms improving once the menstrual flow begins or increases in volume. The pulse is typically wiry. The tongue color is purplish, darkish, or normal with a normal thin coating.

Disease Mechanism: The Liver is the tempermental Organ. If one experiences unrelieved stress or frustration, Liver Qi will be unable to flow smoothly, and the subjective experience of this is depression, irritability, or anxiety. If the Qi flow is not smooth or

57

if the Qi is trapped in the upper body it may affect the breasts, flanks, ribs, or upper back. The frequent sighing is the attempt of the woman to relieve this pent up Qi. The patency or smoothe and even flow of the Liver Qi and the flow of Qi over the *Ren* channel control the timing and regularity of the menstruation. If either or both lose their patency, the menstrual cycle may become irregular. The impatent Liver energy may also disrupt other functions in the lower part of the body, either causing the Large Intestine to become irregular and unsmooth (constipation), or causing distention and pain (pre-menstrual bloating) in the lower abdomen. The wiry pulse is a sign that the energy is Stagnated, as is the darkish tongue body.

2. Depressive Liver Fire and Stomach Fire

Signs and Symptoms: These are similar to those listed above with the addition that the breast distention may now become more painful and there is more likely to be lumps which do not disappear with the onset of the period, or mastitis if the woman is nursing (*Ru Yong* described above); a bloody or yellow discharge from the nipple; a bitter taste in the mouth; a red tongue body; irascibility; chest oppression or stuffiness; a fast and wiry pulse; cold hands and feet; foul breath; recurrent toothaches or sores in the mouth. There may be a huge appetite or a tendency to nausea after eating.

Disease Mechanism: Qi as an entity is warm. Since life is warm and the body is warm, if enough *Qi* gets stuck in one place, eventually it will become Hot. Also, as mentioned above, "the five emotions transform to Fire". The combination of stuck *Qi* and the related or resultant frustration, depression, etc., if not resolved, will easily transform from Stagnant Qi to Stagnant Fire. This causes the fast quality along with the wiry quality in the pulse, the redness of the tongue, and the bitter taste in the mouth, especially upon arising in the morning. This Heat is a Stagnant Heat, and does not circulate in the body, but remains stuck in the Middle, hence the extremities remain cold, especially in situations of stress. When the Liver gets Hot, it may vent this Heat laterally in the

58

torso, affecting the Stomach due to their close relationship. A Hot Stomach manifests as foul breath, toothache, mouth sores, and an incessant uncomfortable hungry sensation.

3. Liver Qi Congestion with Spleen Deficiency

Signs and Symptoms: All the signs and symptoms listed in #1 plus fatigue; diarrhea; decline in appetite or a craving for sweets; nausea; abdominal distention; possible clear discharge from the breast; cold hands and feet; water retention. The pulse is typically wiry and fine, the tongue pale and puffy with a thin white coating.

Disease Mechanism: If the Liver Qi cannot spread out in its normal physiological way, it is possible for it to disrupt the normal functioning of a number of the other Organs, as seen in #2 above. If the Liver disturbs the Spleen function, symptoms indicating digestive dysfunction (diarrhea, loss of appetite, craving for sweets) may arise. Since the Spleen is the major Organ involved in the creation of Blood and energy (Qi) in the body, the additional symptoms such as fatigue (Qi Deficiency) and pale tongue, scant menstrual blood (Blood Deficiency) can develop. The Deficient Qi will also be unable to hold the fluids within the body properly, accounting for the clear discharge from the breasts.

4. Liver Qi Congestion with Liver Blood Kidney Yin Deficiency

Signs and Symptoms: Premenstrual breast distention; chest oppression; sore lower back; weak lower limbs; general low sexual appetite. The patient may have had a late menarche (over 16 yrs.). The tongue is pale with scant fur; and the pulse is usually fine, deep, and wiry. There may also be dizziness, or light-headed sensations when standing up from a recumbent position; ringing in the ears; dream-disturbed sleep or insomnia; night sweats; flushing cheeks or slight fever in the afternoons; withered or pale complexion.

Disease Mechanism: The Kidneys are housed in the lumbus and are responsible for the strength of the knees and the sexual functions. If the Kidneys become weak the low back and knees may feel weak or sore. If specifically the Yin energy of the Kidneys is weak it will not be able to balance the Yang energy of the Kidneys. This Yang energy will float, causing flushed cheeks and low-grade fever. In Chinese medicine the Kidneys are the Mother of the Liver.⁴⁴ If the Yin (Water) of the Kidneys becomes weak, over time the Blood of the Liver will become weak. If the Liver Blood is weak it will be unable to keep the *Qi* of the Liver rooted and smoothly flowing, leading to dizziness and ringing in the ears. Additionally, the Liver Blood is responsible for housing or storing the Psyche (*Hun*). If the Blood in the Liver becomes weak, this function is not performed, causing the sleep to be disturbed.

5. Liver Qi Congestion with Blood Deficiency

Signs and Symptoms: Same as Liver Qi above plus pale complexion, fatigue, lengthened menstrual cycle, or scant discharge pale in color. The tongue may be pale purple or pale brownish with scant fur and the pulse is typically thready and wiry.

Disease Mechanism: The mechanisms here are similar to those described in #4.

6. Liver Qi Congestion with Liver Blood and Kidney Yang Deficiency

Signs and Symptoms: Breast distention, sore lower back, fatigue, possible loss of sex drive, and a cold feeling in the lower abdomen, pale tongue with a normal coating, pulse thready and slow.

Disease Mechanism: The Yang energy of the Kidneys is the source of all the correct or appropriate Heat in the body. It is possible that constitutionally a woman may have weak Kidney Yang as well as Liver Qi Congestion. The slow quality of the pulse, and the pale tongue reflect this lack of Righteous (the body's normal) Heat, since a Cold situation will slow down the normal flow of Qi and Blood in the body. Additionally, since Righteous Heat is nothing more that enough Qi in one place to make things warm, the lack of Heat indicates a Deficiency of Qi which is seen by the fatigue. Sexual desire is a function of Kidney Yang.

7. Liver Qi with Fire Flaring

Signs and Symptoms: Intense breast pain, as in mastitis; dry mouth; headache in the occiput or vertex area; sudden tinnitus (ringing in the ears); bitter taste in the mouth; flank pain; increased irritability or outbursts of anger; possibly a turbid, yellow vaginal discharge or inflammation of the genitalia; yellow or bloody discharge from the nipple. The tongue is red with yellow fur. The pulse will generally be wiry and fast.

Disease Mechanism: Heat causes pain, and more intense Heat, i.e. Fire, causes more intense pain. Fire evaporates liquids in the body, causing thirst, and speeds up the flow of the Blood, causing the fast pulse and the red tongue. Body secretions tend to become yellow and thick in Fire situations, and mucuous membrane areas such as the vagina, oral, or nasal cavities may become inflammed and sore. The stronger the Fire, the more likely it is that frustration or irritability will then become irascability and outbursts of anger, as the Heat rises. Rising Liver Fire also may manifest as headaches or sudden ringing in the ears.

Aside from constitutional tendencies which bring about the variations on the main theme of these seven patterns, the underlying theme of Liver Qi Congestion is the same in all seven. The differences arise in response to which Organ(s) are stronger or weaker in different people and therefore which way the Liver Qi develops over time in relationship to those other Organs. One can see that most of the signs and symptoms listed are parts of the common PMS constellation. For a fuller discussion of PMS as a disease in itself I refer readers again to Bob Flaws' *Free and Easy: Traditional Chinese Gynecology for American*

Women.

At this point the reader should have a fairly complete idea about the Chinese categorization of breast diseases, their causes and development, and how they are connected to each other. The next step is to explain what can be done to treat breast diseases once they have arisen, and more importantly, to give readers three "free therapies" which they can use on their own to avoid serious breast disease altogether.

SECTION III

The Treatment Of
Breast Disorders

Introduction

Breast disease can be treated *and* it can be prevented. There are Chinese medical treatment plans for all the above mentioned patterns, *Zheng*, and named diseases, *Bing*. These treatments involve Chinese herbs or acupuncture therapy which must be administered professionally. However, in the Tang dynasty (circa 700 CE) there was a famous Chinese physician named Sun Si-miao who said that first one should adjust the patient's diet and lifestyle. If that failed to effect a cure, only then should other treatment be given. Therefore, three important aspects of the therapy for breast diseases and most other types of gynecological disorders as well, are in the hands of the woman herself. These three "free" therapies will help keep a woman healthy and free of symptoms. They are based on simple common sense and can form the basis of *anyone's* health regime or lifestyle. They can be practiced throughout one's life, free of charge.

CHAPTER I

Daily Relaxation

The single most important part of any treatment program for Stagnation of Liver Qi is daily relaxation. This therapy, if done consistently and with perseverance can make a difference on a longterm basis, not only in terms of symptoms, but on the fundamental level of who a person is. The reason this therapy is so effective is that it addresses the longterm effects of stress and emotional upset, which are at the root of all problems due to Liver Qi Stagnation. In most cases having an emotional component, I believe this therapy can be as or even more beneficial than a good deal of the currently available psychotherapy. Please do not misunderstand. I have personally experienced useful psychotherapic work, and sometimes may recommend both psychotherapy and daily relaxation to a client. However, *many* forms of "talk" therapy allow or even foster the patient going over and over and over their problems, both real and fabricated, in such as way as to foster the continuation of the same types of thought patterns over and over and over again. This does not eradicate the problem, nor does it often deal with the person's real problems at all. I am not anti-psychotherapy in all cases, but I also believe that whatever happened that makes one frustrated or angry is better released in one moment and forgotten in the next. One can do little about the traffic, or one's mother's manipulative behavior when one was a child, or the fact that the boss was is a bad mood this morning. Better to let go the emotions as much as possible and do what needs to be done in one's life. That may include moving away from where mother lives or changing jobs. Holding onto the anger and frustration is not useful and we have demonstrated that it is deleterious to the health. Regular daily programmed relaxation will help anyone to do the necessary letting go.

In our culture stress is endemic -- job stress, political stress, environmental pollution stress, relationship stress, sexual stress, nuclear warfare stress, the stress of the constant decisions required by living in a "free" society. We have created a society which produces more stress than the human body can process and still remain healthy. Past a certain age, most of us will develop symptoms due to this fact. These symptoms may come and go and we can learn to keep them largely under control, but it is arrogant and unreasonable to think that we can forever keep up the often frenetic pace (physically or emotionally) which many of us must in order to survive and still be free of the ravages of stress.

Women especially find themselves at a time and place in history with "unlimited" options, where our roles are multiple and our sense of self often ill-defined. Our family structure is weaker and less supportive than at any time in American history; community support for parenting is inadequate; divorce is endemic; and the stay-at-home mother-and-housewife is no longer an option in most cases. The sexual confusion wrought by the '60s and '70s is even worse with the arrival of life-threatening sexually transmitted diseases. The constant demands on the time of the average 35-40 year-old woman in our society often leave us with no "down" time and the feeling of being always behind, always pushed, always squeezed.

Daily relaxation therapy is one way to turn off the Heat of stress, loosen the vise grip of that squeezed feeling, and lessen the toll that any pressures in our lifestyle can take on our health.

In order for this therapy to have measurable clinical effectiveness there are a few criteria which must be met.

   1. It must result in somatic, physical relaxation as well as

mental relaxation.

2. It must result in the center of consciousness coming out of one's head and into some part of the lower body, preferrably the area of the lower abdomen.

3. It must be done a minimum of 20 minutes per day, although no longer than 30 minutes are required.

4. It must be done every day without missing a single day for at *least* 100 days.

There are many possible techniques which will accomplish this type of relaxation, including hatha yoga, meditation, biofeedback, etc. The easiest way, however, is to purchase one or two relaxation or stress reduction tapes available at healthfood stores, "new age" bookstores, etc. These take about 25-30 minutes each, are relatively inexpensive and require minimal discipline.

Some people say that they cannot relax, or that it is very difficult for them to keep their mind concentrated during meditation, or that they do not have time to relax. It is precisely these people who need to relax the most. The tapes are helpful for these people, in that, to some extent, they supply the needed concentration. Each time the mind wanders, the tape brings one back to the task at hand, so that one does not need to concentrate on anything, just to listen to the tape.

Additionally, it is best to try to do the tape at the same time each day, so that after a while it becomes like eating, getting dressed, or brushing your teeth, i.e. a nondiscretionary part of your day.

At the end of three months a person may expect to be calmer, less flappable, and have a generally increased state of health with fewer of their prior symptoms manifesting.[45] At the end of three years of regular practice, one will be a different person altogether.

CHAPTER II

Regular Exercise

In order to be effective for Liver Qi Stagnation, exercise must be of an aerobic nature. That means it must increase the heart rate and respiration to close to double of the resting rate and keep it there for at least 20 minutes. Like the relaxation, no further health gains are made after 30 minutes. This may be fulfilled by any one of a number of activities or sports. Whatever exercise you can find that keeps your interest is satisfactory, but it must be done regularly, at least every other day.

This has three main functions.

> 1. Aerobic exercise strengthens the Lungs, which in Chinese medicine are responsible for holding the Liver in check.

> 2. It releases any type of Stagnation, and circulates pent up Liver Qi, sort of like venting steam from a pressure cooker.

> 3. It increases Spleen activity, improving appetite and elimination, boosting the overall energy of the body by increasing the Spleen's production of Qi and Blood. When the Spleen is strong, there is less

likelihood that Dampness and Phlegm will be produced, which we have seen is very important in preventing breast disease.

One of my clients recently reported that her chronic premenstrual breast distention is greatly reduced since she began regular aerobic exercise. Her report is not surprising. While exercise may not eradicate the root cause of breast diseases -- stress and emotional imbalance -- when combined with daily relaxation it is very effective at coping with stress and circulating Stagnant Qi. It is therefore an important part of preventive treatment and should not be overlooked.

CHAPTER III

Dietary Adjustments

Because the single most important cause of breast disorders is related to the emotional life of a woman, diet is not their single most important therapy. However, right diet is an important supporting therapy and unless some dietary adjustments are made, it will be difficult for most women to remain as healthy as possible.

In order to treat the Liver through dietary therapy, there are two approaches, one direct and one indirect. The direct approach is to avoid foods which aggravate the Liver. The indirect method is to eat a diet which supports the Stomach and Spleen. This is a classically accepted method of treatment for Liver disorders even when using herbal or acupuncture therapy.[46] The list of foods which are best to avoid by people suffering from Chinese Liver disorders includes:

-coffee, and other caffeinated foods and beverages

-alcohol, except in small, infrequent amounts

-greasy, fried or oily foods

-spicy, pungent, hot dishes such as curries or chilies

-meat and hard to digest foods

71

-smoking

-recreational drugs

Most women with breast lumps or pain are aware of the connection between foods which contain xanthines (coffee, black teas, colas, chocolate) and the exacerbation of their symptoms. Chinese medicine considers these substances to be drugs, not foods. As such their functions are to strongly activate the Qi, and bring the energy from the core of the body to the surface. In the process of doing this some Blood and Yin (substance and fluid) are lost from the body, which skews the relationship between the Blood and Qi, Yin and Yang, even further than it was before ingesting the caffeine (xanthines). Of course most women with Liver Qi Stagnation will like the "kick" which the caffeine gives to the stuck Qi. There is some movement caused by the caffeine which, for a little while, frees up the flow of the Qi. However, because the Liver must be kept nourished by Blood in order for its Qi to move smoothely and patently, the net effect is that the caffeine, by wasting the Liver Blood, leaves the Liver less able to promote free flow of the Qi. Of any dietary recommendations, eschewing coffee and other caffeine substances altogether is probably the single most important.

Alcohol, when used only occasionally, has the ability to relax the whole body and is considered to be useful for certain people in certain situations. However, alcohol has a Damp Hot energy. When used regularly it will tend to overheat the Liver and Stomach and dampen the Spleen. We have seen above how Liver Heat and Spleen Dampness are such important issues in breast disease. Jin Zi-jiu, a famous nineteenth century physician, in the *Jin Zi-jiu Zhuan Ji (Jin Zi-jiu's Medical Contemplations)* states,

> "Alcohol has a volatile nature which damages the
> Spirit and injures the Blood. Its energy is Hot and
> it leads to waste and decline. Alcohol first enters
> the Gallbladder-Liver where Gallbladder Fire first
> explodes. The *Qi* loses its restraint and
> descension....The Blood bcomes unsettled and as

72

a result, rebellious ascension with vomiting of blood can occur. Moreover, alcohol is Damp as well as Hot. Dampness injures the Spleen. This creates Stagnant Food and Phlegm which easily overstuffs the *Qi* Mechanism. In short...drinking injures the Blood."[47]

In relationship to breast disease, it is the Liver Qi which is Excessive and not free flowing. It is the Liver Blood which keeps Liver Qi relaxed, smooth, and free flowing. Therefore, similarly to caffeine, it is important to limit or curtail alcohol consumption in order not to waste or injure the Blood.

Greasy, heavy, difficult to digest foods likewise tend to produce Dampness, clogging the digestive tract and creating Food Stagnation which exacerbates an already Stagnated situation. Additionally, it is the Liver/Gall Bladder which are responsible for the creation/secretion of bile which must work to digest all fats. Overconsumption of greasy foods creates more work for the Liver, tending to depress it further.

Meat is fine in small quantities if well cooked, and eaten only a few times per week. In fact, people who have grown up eating meat seem to be healthier in the long run if they continue to eat a small amount on a regular basis. Longterm vegetarianism in such people tends to produce Qi and Blood Deficiency which is difficult to address in any other way than to reintroduce small quantities of meat and meat broths into the diet. I have even seen a case where a woman's breast disease went from benign to malignant due to a raw foods and strict vegetarian regime. Rather than shrink her tumor, it only grew faster due to her Stagnation being so aggravated by Qi and Blood Deficiency. Soups made with meat broths or marrow bones are an excellent way to get the most nourishment from the meat without ingesting the parts which are harder to digest and more deleterious to the body.

Spicy and pungent foods have a similar effect to that of caffeine. They have a tendency to move the Qi and therefore create an initial burst of energy, but their net effect is to further imbalance the

73

Liver by weakening the Lungs (whose job it is to keep the Liver in check), making the Liver Hot, aggravating the entire situation and making it even more complicated to treat. In the *Nei Jing*, one of Chinese medicine's earliest and most important classics, it is said that pungent food is forbidden in all Qi diseases.

Tobacco has a Dry, Bitter energy which damages the Qi and attacks the Lungs. Again, it is the Lungs which, according to Chinese physiology, must keep the Liver under control. If the Lungs are weakened, the Liver will become too strong. The Lungs are also the Mother of the Kidney[44], and it is the Kidney Water which keeps the Liver nourished and moist, free from pathogenic Heat.

There are many types of recreational drugs and they will have varying effects on the body. In general, however, all those which have the effect of producing a "high", or making the body feel more energized, are extremely deleterious to the body, especially the Kidneys. Drugs such as amphetamines, cocaine, and all psychotropic drugs, create that feeling of extra energy or "high" by using the *Jing* or Essence from the Kidneys. This Essence is brought up through the various layers of the body by the action of the drug, creating excitation and energy as it passes through each layer. When it reaches the Surface, however, it evaporates off the Surface and is gone. *Jing* Essence is the deepest level of energy in the body, and is very difficult to replace. The Kidneys are like the Fort Knox of the body, and the *Jing* is like gold. Once used, this gold may require years to be replaced. Recreational drugs, then, will speed up the aging process by weakening the Kidneys. Since the Kidneys are the ultimate source of normal or Righteous (healthy) Fire and Water in the body, longterm weakness of the Kidneys eventually affects the energy and balance among all the Organs.

Additionally, as the source of all Righteous Heat in the body, the Kidney is the pilot light for the cooking process of digestion. If the Kidney becomes weak this often leads to a weakening of the digestion, i.e. the Stomach/Spleen. If this pair becomes weak or imbalanced, we have already discussed the possible negative consequences which may arise -- depressed creation of new Qi and

74

Blood, and the accumulation of Dampness and Phlegm.

According to the *Nei Jing*, the first rule in treating Liver disease is to support preventively the Stomach/Spleen. Based on Five phase theory, the Liver "controls" these two Organs. Therefore, when the Liver becomes Excess, they become weak. By keeping these two strong, however, the Liver can be indirectly kept in check and there are goods one *can* eat which support the Stomach/Spleen. These include:

-eating foods which are cooked and warm

-eating foods which are easily digestible

-eating mostly grains, vegetables, meat broths

-avoiding cold, frozen, and raw foods, or keeping the quantities of these foods small in the overall diet

-avoiding foods which produce Dampness such as milk products *if* there is copious mucous production

-the cautious usage of warming spices such as ginger, cardamom, nutmeg, cinnamon

If one considers that the Stomach is like a cooking pot which must make everything which is ingested into 100 degree "soup" before it can be further digested, one can understand the dictum concerning cooked and easily digestible foods. Anything which pre-digests the food for the Stomach will ease its work and allow it to function well. Consider that one does not give raw foods to a sick person or a small baby. To help someone who is sick to recover one gives them the most easily digestible foods, which support the job of the Stomach. Among traditional peoples living in temperate climates the most common diet largely consisted of well-cooked grains and fresh, *but cooked* vegetables, and a small amount of meats or meat broths. Even such "modern" diets as the Pritikin diet are based on this idea.

There are some schools of thought which say that cooking destroys vitamins. What these people fail to understand is the difference between gross and net. A raw carrot may have more vitamins than a cooked one if measured in a laboratory *outside the Stomach*. However, if a raw carrot has, let's say, 100 units of vitamin A and a cooked one has only 50 units, but the Stomach can absorb 40 units from the cooked one and only 20 from the raw one, which one has a better net effect? What happens on a laboratory countertop has nothing to do with the process of digestion inside the body. The body can absorb nutrients from cooked food much more efficiently than it can from raw.

While small amounts may not cause any problem in most people, dairy products are known to cause the production of Dampness in the body when eaten to excess. Pathogenic accumulations of Dampness lower or interfere with Spleen function, hence causing the production of Phlegm. If Spleen function needs to be supported to avoid the production of Dampness and Phlegm, foods such as dairy, which tend to be difficult for the Spleen to Transform properly should be eaten in moderation.

Frozen foods such as ice cream and frozen soy products are even harder for the Stomach/Spleen to process than dairy products and are probably one of the worst inventions of humankind. Consider that up until 40 or 50 years ago it was impossible to have frozen foods at all. While refrigeration may be a boon to us in many ways, we need to learn to use it more judiciously. Ingesting frozen foods requires the Stomach and Spleen to expend a great deal of energy just to get the food up to a temperature at which it can be digested. This is a great waste of Qi and over time will weaken the Spleen, again causing an accumulation of Dampness and Phlegm.

Warming spices such as nutmeg, cardomom, cinnamon, ginger, etc. may be eaten to good advantage in small amounts as long as there are no signs of Stomach Heat (see the patterns of disharmony listed on pages 60-61 for these symptoms). They will tend to give a mild boost to Qi movement, without the damaging and imbalancing effects of caffeine or heavy spicy foods. They can be included in the diet in judicious amounts.

CHAPTER IV

Professional Therapies

While all these self-therapies are useful and will improve the situation of any woman experiencing breast pain, distention, or lumps, they may not be enough. If symptoms persist, or if lumps are already present, professionally administered therapies may be necessary for quicker and greater longterm remission of symptoms. Here let me say again that successful treatment can take place at any point in this process, no matter what the symptoms, if a woman has the motivation and will.

Professionally administered Chinese medicine is definitely effective in the treatment of the majority of breast diseases. Several recent studies available in acupuncture and Chinese medical journals show excellent results in the treatment of breast neoplasms with the use of acupuncture or Chinese herbal medicine. In a study of 500 cases of hyperplasia (lumps) of the breast treated by acupuncture, there was a 95.71% effective rate with only one course of 10 treatments. These results were better than the control group which was treated with a combination of Chinese herbal medicine and Western drug therapy.[48] In another experimental study on mice with breast tumors, a combination of radiation therapy and moxibustion[49] was used. The group of mice treated with this combination of therapies showed the longest survival rate of the four different groups tested.[50] Most American practitioners will want to administer a combination of both herbal and acupuncture therapy, although either may be effective depending upon the case.

Although each individual case is different, as a general rule acupuncture is most effective in treating Qi disorders, especially those which involve the mind and emotions, and in reducing pain. Herbal therapies are more effective in treating the Blood level of energy and in supplementing Deficiencies of all types in the body. However, both acupuncture and Chinese herbal medicine treat Qi, Blood, Food, Damp, Phlegm, and Fire Stagnations. When both acupuncture and herbal medicine are used in tandem for the treatment of breast diseases, the acupuncture acts as a strong, local, and external stimulus while the herbs work gently and continuously from the inside. But, no matter which type of therapy is used, most patients should expect that for therapy to be successful, it will require *at least* one month for each year that they have experienced the problem.

If a woman has developed breast cancer, probably the best treatment is a combination of traditional Chinese and modern Western medicines. By the time a woman's imbalance has degenerated to cancer, traditional Chinese medicine by itself may not be fast enough. Western medicine, although heroic and quick, often also causes many side-effects and complications. But, these complications can usually be treated very well with Chinese medicine. But, the complications can usually be treated very well with Chinese medicine. These days, more and more patients and physicians alike are opting for lumpectomies whenever possible followed by radiation and/or chemotherapy. Chinese medicine can be taken before radiation to minimize it negative effect. It can also be taken during and after radiation and chemotherapy to minimize and treat their side-effects quite effectively, including nausea, fatigue, anemia, and even hair loss. *The Treatment of Cancer by Integrated Chinese-Western Medicine* by Zhang Dai-zhao presents a very clear, step by step methodology for combining Chinese and Western medicines in the treatment of breast cancer.[51]

Women who have already been treated by Western medicine alone for breast cancer should also consider that Western medicine

78

rarely treats the underlying energetic reason for the development of cancer in the first place. This underlying cause persists after surgery, radiation, and chemotherapy and this explains why cancer often recurs. These heroic and swift therapies may give a woman a much needed respite, but she should not be fooled into thinking that they have aborted the energetic process at the root of her problem. However, traditional Chinese medicine can identify and treat these root causes. Such treatment usually is a life-time process. As Dr. Zhang says,

> ...perseverance in prolonged and active integrated therapy is one important step to consolidate and enhance the therapeutic effect and prevent recurrence. Malignant tumors are characterized by their rapid growth and their tendency to reoccur and metastasize. Due to the fact that there is no satisfactory radical therapy for late stage cancers, it is more important that doctors assume a responsible attitude in order to maintain a long-term relationship and to offer (their) knowledge of preventing and treating cancerous conditions, thus encouraging patients to continue long-term treatment. It should never be assumed that when the symptoms are relieved after treatments such as surgery, radiation, chemotherapy, or the internal ingestion of herbal ingredients for a period of time that the cancerous condition has been (completely) corrected and that therapy should be suspended.[52]

In order to find a qualified Chinese medical practitioner, one can contact state acupuncture associations, local acupuncture/Chinese medicine schools, the National Commission for the Certification of Acupuncturists[53], or the American Association of Acupuncture and Oriental Medicine[54]. Be sure to ask each practitioner contacted what their educational background is and if they have ever treated your particular problem and with what success.

Conclusion

According to the tenets of Chinese medical theory, minor breast disorders should not be left untreated, nor are they unavoidable discomforts of womanhood. Even the presence of simple breast tenderness before the period is a symptom of minor imbalance which can and should be corrected or improved.

By treating these simple disorders effectively, a woman can help herself avoid more serious ones in later years. The occurrence of such problems as dysfunctional uterine bleeding, uterine fibroids, debilitating premenstrual syndrome, certain types of infertility, endometriosis, menopausal syndrome, and breast tumors both malignant and benign, are all related to this same continuum of imbalance and can all be lessened or eliminated by traditional Chinese medicine. By treating any of these, one also is preventing the arisal of serious disorders in all other related parts of their body.

It is my hope that through the insights and wisdom of Chinese medicine presented in this small book, the pain and suffering of many women may be lessened or eliminated. For *most* breast diseases it is certain that Chinese medicine offers a logical, rational description of their nature and progression, and effective therapies for their treatment. More importantly, the treatments for these imbalances put a great deal of power and control directly in the hands of women themselves, which is perhaps the greatest gift we are offering with this publication.

ENDNOTES

1   Al-Khafaji, Mazin, "The Differentiation and Treatment of Mammary Dysplasia and Fibroadenoma by Chinese Medicine", *Journal of Chinese Medicine*, UK, #28, September, 1988

2   "The idea of Qi is fundamental to Chinese medical thinking, yet no one English word or phrase can adequately capture its meaning. We can say that everything in the universe, organic and inorganic, is composed of and defined by its Qi. But Qi is not some primordial, immutable material, nor is it merely vital energt, although the word is occasionally so translated. Chinese thought does not distinguish between matter and energy, but we can perhaps think of Qi as matter on the verge of becoming energy, or energy at the point of materializing. To Chinese though, however, such discussion of what a concept means in itself - a discussion that the Western mind expects in any systematic exposition - is completely foreign. Neither the classical nor modern Chinese texts speculate on the nature of Qi, nor do they attempt to conceptualize it. Rather, Qi is perceived functionally - by what it does."
Kaptchuk, Ted, *The Web That Has No Weaver*, Congdon & Weed, NY, 1983, p. 35-36

3   *Webster's 7th New Collegiate Dictionary*, G. & C. Merriam Co., Springfield, MA, 1967, p. 396

4   Cooper, Patricia, ed., *Better Homes & Gardens Women's Health and Medical Guide,* Meredith Corporation, Publisher, Des Moines, IA, 1981, p.542

5   Lauerson, N.H., & Stukane, E., *PMS: PMS And You,* Simon & Shuster, Inc., NY, 1983, p. 118

6   Cooper, Patricia, ed., op. cit., p. 546

7   Berkow, Robert, & Talbott, John, ed., *The Merck Manual of Diagnosis and Therapy*, Merck, Sharp, & Dohme Research Labs, Rahway, NJ, 1977, p. 971

8   Ibid., p. 971

9   Shell, E.R., "Your Best Breast Defense", *Mlle Magazine*, May, 1987, p. 248

10 Cooke, Dr. Cynthia W., & Dworkin, Susan, *The Ms Guide to a Woman's Health*, Anchor Press/Doubleday, Garden City, NY, 1979, p. 358

11 Anon., "Healthfront: Painful Breasts May Benefit From Iodine", *Prevention Magazine*, April, 1987, p. 12

12 Cooke, C.W., & Dworkin, S., op.cit. p. 358

13 Berkow, R., & Talbott, J., op. cit., p. 970

14 Ibid., p.972

15 Anon., *The Breast Cancer Digest*, U.S. Department of Health and Human Services, 1988, p. 2

16 Berkow, R., & Talbott, J. op. cit., p. 972

17 Anon., *What You Need To Know About Breast Cancer*, U.S. Department of Health & Human Services, 1988, p. 10-11

18 Ibid., p. 22-23

19 Shell, E.R., op. cit., p.246

20 Because the *Chinese* medical definitions of the Organs is functional and energetic, as opposed to strictly material, the author would discourage readers from purchasing any over the counter medicines described as being good for

84

conditions of the *Western* organs. If any reader feels that they have an imbalance in an Organ similar to what is described in this book for which they desire treatment, we suggest that they seek out a professional practitioner of traditional Chinese medicine. See footnotes #53 and 54

21   Larre, Claude, Schatz, Jean, & Rochat de la Valle, Elizabeth, *Survey of Traditional Chinese Medicine*, Institut Ricci, Paris, 1986

22   Kaptchuk, Ted, op.cit., P.223

23   Liu Yanchi, *The Essential Book of Traditional Chinese Medicine*, Vol. I, Columbia University Press, NY, 1988, p.77

24   *Chinese-English Terminology of Traditional Chinese Medicine*, Hunan Science & Technology Press, Hunan Province, People's Republic of China, 1981, p. 115

25   Flaws, Bob, "Premenstrual Breast Distention", *Free and Easy: Traditional Chinese Gynecology for American Women*, Blue Poppy Press, Boulder, CO, 1986, p. 104

26   Gu Shi, *Yong Yi Da Quan*, quoted by Al-Khafaji, Mazin, op. cit., p.8

27   Chen Jirui & Wang, Nissi, *Acupuncture Case Histories From China*, Eastland Press, Seattle, WA, 1988, p.257

28   Al-Khafaji, Mazin, op. cit., p. 8

29   Flaws, Bob, op. cit., p. 104

30   Ibid., p. 97

31   Ibid., p. 97

32   Zhejiang College of Traditional Chinese Medicine, Zhang,

Ting-liang, trans., *A Handbook of Traditional Chinese Gynecology*, Blue Poppy Press, Boulder CO, 1987, p. 119

33   Jia Kun, *Carcinoma*, The Commercial Press, Hong Kong, 1985, p. 98

34   This list of patterns associated with breast cancer is a compilation from several sources including *The Treatment of Cancer By Intregrated Chinese-Western Medicine, Carcinoma, Treating Cancer with Chinese Herbs.*

35   Zhang, Dai-zhao, *The Treatment of Cancer By Integrated Chinese-Western Medicine*, Blue Poppy Press, Boulder, CO, 1989, p. 18

36   Jia Kun, op. cit., p. 98

37   Hsu, H.Y., *Treating Cancer With Chinese Herbs*, OHAI, Los Angeles, 1982, p. 82

38   Zhang, Dai-zhao, op. cit., p. 81-83

39   Wilkinson, J.F., *Don't Raise Your Child To Be A Fat Adult*, The Bobbs-Merril Co., Inc., NY, 1980, p. 18

40   *Essentials of Conformation in Chinese Medicine* and *Terminology of Chinese Medicine*, as quoted by Hsu, H.Y., op. cit., p. 83-84

41   Flaws, Bob, op. cit., p. 98-99

42   Al-Khafaji, Mazin, op.cit., p.8-10

43   Plum Seed Qi is the Chinese name for a condition in which one has the sensation of a lump in the throat which can neither be swallowed nor coughed up. It is considered to be a manifestion of Liver Qi Congestion, and it may or may

not involve Stagnant Phlegm as well.

44   One of the major historical theories of Chinese medicine is the so-called Five Element or Five Phase cycle. Each major Organ is associated with an Element: Wood (Liver), Fire (Heart), Earth (Spleen), Metal (Lung), Water (Kidney). It is said that each Element "produces" the next in this order, hence the idea of one Element, and therefore one Organ, being the Mother of the next. I refer interested readers to *Five Elements and Ten Stems* by Kiiko Matsumoto and Stephen Birch.

45   Benson, Herbert, *The Relaxation Response*, G.K. Hall & Co., Boston, 1976, p.86-87

46   Lee, Miriam, *Clinical Applications of St. 36, Sp. 6, C. 4 and 11 and Lung 7: One Combination of Points Can Treat Many Diseases*, self-published, Palo Alto, CA, p. 70

47   Jin Zi-jiu, *Jin Zi-jiu Zhang Ji (Jin Zi-jiu's Medical Contemplations)*, trans. by Michael Helme, *Timing and The Times*, Flaws, B., Chace, C., & Helme, M., Blue Poppy Press, Boulder, CO, 1986, p. 128

48   Chang, Yung-hsien, Haw, Dou-mong, and Hung, Yu-tse, "Effect of Irradiation and Moxibustion on Mice Bearing Breast Tumors", *Fourth International Congress of Chinese Medicine,* University of San Francisco, CA, July 29-31, 1988.

49   Moxibustion is a treatment procedure in Chinese medicine whereby an herbal ingredient, Artemesia vulgaris sinensis, is burned over, under, on, or around an acupuncture point. This therapy is usually used to warm and tonify the Organ or channel being treated.

50   Guo Chengjie, "Effects of Acupuncture in the Treatment

of 500 Cases of Hyperplasia of Breast", *Chinese Acupuncture & Moxibustion*, Vol. 6, No.4, August, 1986, pp.2-4

51   Zhang Dai-zhao, *The Treatment of Cancer by Integrated Chinese-Western Medicine*, trans. by Zhang Ting-liang & Bob Flaws, Blue Poppy Press, Boulder, CO, 1988

52   Ibid., p. 135-136

53   National Commission for the Certification of Acupuncturists, 1424 16th St. NW Suite 105, Washington, D.C. 20036, 202/232-1404

54   American Association of Acupuncture and Oriental Medicine regional offices: Florida 813-541-2666; Maryland 301-652-2828; Minnesota 612-925-4639; California 415-449-4327; New York 212-682-8149; Seattle 206-323-8940